THE DIETITIAN PRESENTS

THE SMART GUIDE TO PLANT-BASED EATING

WELL-PLANNED MEALS MADE EASY
+ RECIPES FOR 28 DAYS

ANNE HOLMES, MS, RDN

Copyright © 2022 by Anne Holmes
All rights reserved.
ISBN 979-8-9850476-0-8 (paperback)

This book is protected by copyright. No part of this book may be used or reproduced in any form without written permission from the copyright owner.

The views and ideas expressed in this book are those of its author. It is intended to provide helpful general information to those interested in plant-based eating. It is not in any way intended to substitute for advice from your physician or qualified healthcare professional which you should consult regarding individual medical conditions, concerns, or changes in diet. Anne Holmes is not your personal dietitian. For personalized medical, health, dietary, or other help and advice, the reader should always consult a personal physician and/or qualified healthcare professional. Never disregard professional medical advice or delay seeking medical treatment because of information you have read in this book or on anneholmesnutrition.com. Any injury, damage, or loss that the reader may experience as a direct or indirect consequence of following any suggestions or directions given in this book or participating in any of the activities described are specifically disclaimed by the author and publisher.

The author's best efforts have been made to provide accurate reference values and internet addresses at the time of publication, and the author disclaims liability from errors made or changes that occurred after publication. Third-party websites and their content are not under the control of the author and the author disclaims all liability arising from their use. Any mention or discussion of products, companies, organizations, or authorities mentioned in this book does not imply endorsement of the author by those entities or vice versa.

Cheerios® cereal and Total® cereal are registered trademarks of General Mills, used with permission. Earth Balance® and Smart Balance® are registered trademarks of Conagra Brands Inc., used with permission. Grape-Nuts® cereal is a registered trademark of Post Consumer Brands, LLC, used with permission. Camilla Brand® is a registered trademark of L.H. Hayward & Co., LLC. Camilla Brand® Lady Cream Peas used with permission. Better Than Bouillon® is a brand of Summit Hill Foods. Better Than Bouillon® bases used with permission. Edward & Sons® is a registered trademark of Edward & Sons Trading Co. Edward & Sons® bouillon cubes used with permission. Follow Your Heart® is a registered trademark of Follow Your Heart®/Earth Island®. Follow Your Heart® Dairy-Free Cheese Parmesan Style used with permission. Tofutti® is a registered trademark of Tofutti Brand, Inc. Tofutti® Better Than Sour Cream used with permission.

Chapter page images by Yuliya Volkovska/ Alamy Stock Vector.

Recipe and food calculations are approximations made by a registered dietitian nutritionist using NutriBase 19 Pro + Edition, v.19.1 (CyberSoft, Inc.), information from food manufacturers, and/or the United States Department of Agriculture (USDA), Agricultural Research Service FoodData Central.

Website: anneholmesnutrition.com

Contents

ACKNOWLEDGMENTS V

PREFACE VII

PART 1: FOUNDATION FOR NUTRITIONAL MEAL PLANNING

    CHAPTER 1: INTRODUCTION 3

    CHAPTER 2: NUTRITION BASICS 5

    CHAPTER 3: MEAL PLANNING FOR A PLANT-BASED DIET 9

    CHAPTER 4: TIPS FOR SUCCESS 13

    CHAPTER 5: PLANNING FOR SNACKS AND DESSERTS 17

    CHAPTER 6: BEVERAGES 21

    CHAPTER 7: PROTEIN MATTERS 25

    CHAPTER 8: NUTRIENTS OF CONCERN AND SUMMARY CHART 31

PART 2: COOKING ESSENTIALS AND RECIPES

    COOKING ESSENTIALS FOR RECIPE SUCCESS 67

    THE RECIPES 73

        SUPPER OR MAIN MEAL 76

        SIDES 139

    Lunch... **152**
    Breakfast **164**
    Beverages **177**
    Desserts **180**

APPENDIX A: ONE WEEK OF SAMPLE MEALS WITH THE WEEKLY MENU PLANNER **185**

APPENDIX B: 28 DAYS OF SAMPLE MEALS AND NUTRIENT INFORMATION **191**

APPENDIX C: RECIPE NUTRIENT ESTIMATIONS:
CALCIUM, VITAMIN D, VITAMIN B12, IODINE, IRON, ZINC, CHOLINE, POTASSIUM, PHOSPHORUS **207**

NOTES **213**

INDEX **225**

Acknowledgments

This book would not have been possible without the help and support of many wonderful people whom I want to thank.

I am deeply indebted to my loving family. First and foremost, I want to acknowledge our beloved uncle, Dr. Ronald Easmann. His editorial skills, thoughts, and support have been constant and crucial throughout the development of this book. I am forever thankful for all of the countless hours he spent diligently helping to refine and shape this book. My wonderful Dad and Mom, Bob and Barbara Anne Bowling, have always been such a powerful source of encouragement for me to reach my goals and dreams. I am so appreciative for all the wisdom they have passed along to me and for giving me the gift of education. Receiving business advice from Dad, and being covered in prayers by Mom were essential ingredients for this book. I would also like to recognize the profound influence that their emphasis on healthy eating has had on me. My dear mother-in-law, Pam Holmes, is amazing! Her meals are always such tasty works of art made with love. Many of the recipes in this book are inspired from Pam's recipes. I am so thankful to her for always supporting me with heartfelt encouragement as well as the latest cooking tools, access to cooking research, and so much more. My sisters, Betsy Duggar and Dr. Ginger Barranco, are awesome sisters who took their time to give me candid advice! My two sons, William and Henry, who are the light of my life, ate all my cooking experiments—tasty and terrible! These fellas have been with me through it all—giving me sweet encouragement, helping me to fulfill my dreams. I hope they follow their dreams to the fullest! Most importantly, my loving husband, Dr. Will Holmes, provided invaluable inspiration, edits, and business advice. I am grateful that he, too, ate all of the meals I tried! Because of his support, I was able to reach my goal of writing this nutrition book.

A very special thanks to all my dear friends. Pam Davis, who with continual good cheer, always listened to me talk about this book, tried out my recipes, and had her family take a beautiful garden picture for me. Kenzie Jardina and Kristen Smith made our writing club such a fun and productive time together. I am forever grateful to Kenzie for assisting me with setting up my website. To my book club (Alyson, Gaby, Grace, Jennifer, Sofia, Yahayra, and Wendy), I cherish the times and meals we've shared.

I would also like to thank Chip Gaskill, Esq., for all his expert legal counsel and the Hamilton Mill Library and staff, especially Noelle Rose, who provided technological assistance.

All praise to God, our sustainer, for giving me such a wonderful family and friends. And . . . here's to taking care of our bodies, God's magnificent creation!

Preface

I was inspired to write *The Smart Guide to Plant-Based Eating* because of my love for and desire to promote the concept of achieving excellent health through healthy eating. As a dietitian, I am frequently asked my opinion on various diets. Many people are confused, frustrated, and overwhelmed by the conflicting recommendations about diet and nutrition that are present in today's popular culture. It is often difficult to respond to questions about diets with simple answers. An individual's diet is influenced by many factors, each of which may vary in importance from person to person. However, the most fundamental requirement of any diet is that it must provide you with the nutrients that your body needs to function and thrive. I want to share a great plan for your meals, based on current principles of sound nutrition, that I can stand behind and recommend.

My plan is flexibly plant-based and employs an approach emphasizing food selection, meal planning, and food preparation practices that are focused on consistently providing the nutrient and energy levels needed for proper bodily function.

The Smart Guide to Plant-Based Eating identifies the nutrient requirements that are most difficult to obtain within plant-based diets and offers menus that include foods containing these substances. It prepares individuals to design their own meals with menus that are focused on nutritional value. *The Smart Guide to Plant-Based Eating* also encourages the meal planner to be mindful of the effects that realities such as taste preferences, social pressures, and other circumstances exert on eating practices.

A 4-week meal planning framework is presented in *The Smart Guide to Plant-Based Eating* with recipes for breakfast, lunch, and supper that are entirely plant-based (no meat, eggs, dairy). Tips for adding animal-based ingredients to individual portions in order to satisfy non-plant-based eaters in your family are also included. This guide adheres to current respected standards of nutrition augmented by my personal experiences.

My personal diet is rich in fruits and vegetables including beans, peas, whole-grains, and nuts. While I eat almost all foods, my favorite meals are plant-based. One of the reasons why I love plant-based eating is because it makes me feel great—I have more energy, and my digestive system runs smoothly. However, I believe that a plant-based diet does not have to be followed strictly or "all of the time" to be beneficial. This flexibility can make life easier and more enjoyable. It may also help promote long-term adherence to a mostly plant-based eating pattern. Lastly, I would add that it is important to follow the advice of your physician to ensure the appropriateness of this or any other meal plan for you and your family.

My formal education in nutrition began at Auburn University where I received a bachelor's degree in Nutrition and Food Science. My master's degree in Clinical Nutrition is from the University of Alabama at Birmingham. I have worked in hospitals as Clinical Dietitian, Clinical Nutrition Manager, and Nutrition Support Team Dietitian. In these roles, I have assisted both children and adults in meeting their nutritional needs. Additionally, I have taught many nutrition classes and independently counseled numerous individuals with guidance that was specific for their nutritional requirements.

Since the birth of our second child, I have spent more time focused on my own family. Being married and the mother of two quickly growing boys has been the most amazing and wonderful experience, and it has given me a chance to develop strategies and plans to address the challenges of feeding a family consistently healthy and delicious meals in a time-conscious way.

In *The Smart Guide to Plant-Based Eating*, I have used my own life experiences, current research-based evidence, and standards from reliable sources to establish nutrient requirements to provide foundational information related to plant-based eating and to evaluate the meal plans and recipes presented. The recipes in this guide have been prepared many times in kitchens, my own as well as others, and they have been rated 10 out of 10 by my tasting sources before being accepted. In conclusion, the recipes, plans, and knowledge gained from this guide will help you discover your path to eating healthy every day.

I hope this book will spark some enthusiasm for taking a little time for nutrition in your life!

Anne Holmes, MS, RDN

Part 1:
Foundation for Nutritional Meal Planning

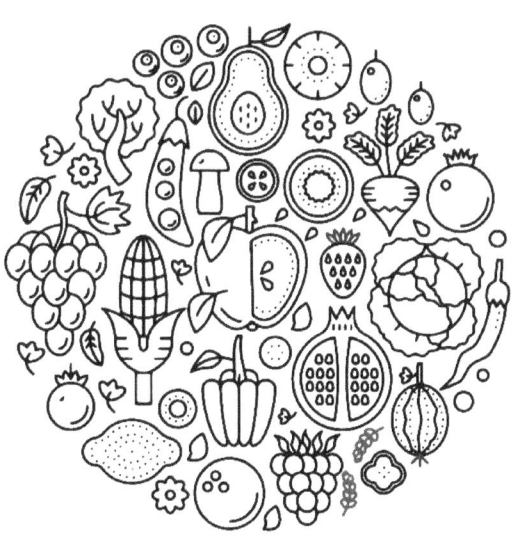

Chapter 1: Introduction

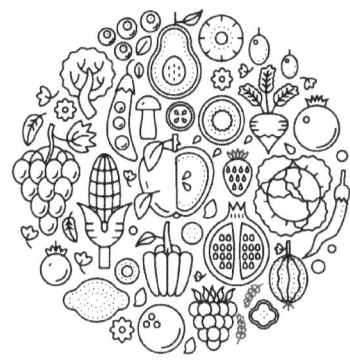

The *Smart Guide to Plant-Based Eating* is a nutritionally focused introduction and guide to plant-based eating that includes a comprehensive meal planning framework with 28 days of recipes for breakfast, lunch, and supper. The recipes are entirely plant-based (no meat, eggs, or dairy). This book is designed to educate and assist anyone who is interested in trying, adopting, or improving their understanding of plant-based eating.

This guide to nutritional eating presents important foundational information about individual nutrients and standards by which the nutritional adequacy of any diet can be assessed. Additional attention is paid to specific elements of plant-based diets which are more likely to lead to nutrient deficiencies. The guide also provides a practical planning framework for nutritionally adequate meals. Finally, the meal planning framework is supported with 4 weeks of plant-based recipes for meals that are healthy, easy to prepare, time conscious, and delicious. By utilizing all three components (nutrition foundation, meal planning, and recipes) you are ready to enjoy the benefits of plant-based eating now and to expand your menus with new recipes in the future. You may decide to follow a plant-based diet "all of the time", "most of the time", or "some of the time" using this book as a guide.

Why plant-based?

Plant-based eating is linked with important health benefits. In particular, persons following plant-based diets have been shown to reduce their risk for type 2 diabetes, heart disease, some cancers, and obesity.[1-12] Evidence suggests that following plant-based eating patterns may slow the progression of chronic kidney disease.[13-14] Additionally, many individuals experience improved digestive health on a plant-based diet. Well-planned plant-based diets are rich in fiber from fruits, vegetables including beans and peas, whole-grains, and nuts. Fiber works together with other phytonutrients to promote a healthy gut microbiome which may reduce inflammatory factors and benefit your immune system.[15-20] High fiber diets also help to normalize bowel function by keeping food particles and toxins moving along in the gut which results in reduced constipation and gas.[21,22]

Why should you use *The Smart Guide to Plant-Based Eating*?

The Smart Guide to Plant-Based Eating takes a refined approach to plant-based dietary patterns. In addition to meeting essential nutrient and energy requirements, the concepts shown in this guide encourage an understanding of nutritional needs, and flexibility to deal with many non-nutritional factors affecting an individual's or entire family's diet.

I think it is important for some groups, especially infants, children, and teens to consume a wider variety of foods. I suggest being flexible. Regularly or occasionally including some animal-based foods in a mostly plant-based diet may help long-term adherence and acceptance. Additional benefits include increased variety in meals and exposure to foods that provide nutrients not plentiful in a purely plant-based diet. However, following a plant-based diet more often than not will increase the likelihood of gaining the long-term health benefits associated with eating a well-planned plant-based diet. Check with your physician prior to beginning a new dietary pattern.

In summary, the information, plans, and recipes presented in this guide will help you chart a course for better nutrition and better health. As each person is different, a plant-based diet may or may not be ideal for you. However, for many people, even those who may be skeptical at first, a plant-based diet as suggested by my guide actually would be a great fit!

Are you interested? If so, grab a garden basket, bowl, or bucket, and let's go fill it with sound nutrition knowledge, flexible and practical meal planning guidelines, and terrific "go-to" recipes and meal ideas that can be used again and again.

Chapter 2: Nutrition Basics

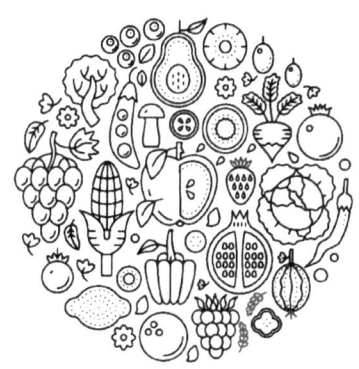

What is a healthy diet?

The basic purpose of any healthy diet is to provide nutrients that supply the variety and quantity of substances necessary to support the energy, structural, and other physiological (functional) processes of your body. Well-planned diets offer appropriate amounts of calories, carbohydrates, proteins, fats, fiber, hydration, vitamins, minerals, and micronutrients. It is essential to select foods that, in combination, will provide these nutritional elements. In addition, food preparation should preserve the nutritional value and promote the edibility of the food that you select.

Plant-based diet

Plant-based refers to the exclusion of all animal products (meat, eggs, dairy) from the diet. A person may follow a plant-based eating pattern to varying degrees (all of the time, most of the time, some of the time). Many people adhere to this pattern of eating as part of their culture, to promote good health, to support a sustainable environment, and/or to encourage animal welfare. The considerations discussed in this book relate to the nutritional and health benefits and concerns related to plant-based eating.

A plant-based diet has two considerations that require special attention when planning meals. One relates to the way in which protein needs are met. The other involves nutrients which may be more challenging to obtain in the recommended quantities from a plant-based diet and includes calcium, vitamin D, vitamin B12, iodine, iron, zinc, choline, and some omega-3 fatty acids. Additionally, anyone following a plant-based diet who has special dietary concerns or may become pregnant should consult with a registered dietitian nutritionist for individual recommendations to meet their needs.

Protein

Every cell in our body contains proteins. Muscle tissue, membranes, bones, skin, hair, nails, body fluids, hormones, antibodies, and many enzymes have protein components.

Proteins are made up of a variety of amino acids which are linked together in complex structures. Amino acids are present in varying types and quantities (as proteins) in most foods. These amino acids are made available by the digestive processes so that your body can use them to make the proteins that it needs.

In addition, the body itself makes some amino acids. Certain amino acids are considered essential, because the body is unable to produce them on its own. Essential amino acids must be taken in through the diet.[1]

Animal-based diets contain major sources of protein in meat (beef, pork, poultry, fish, seafood), eggs, and dairy (milk, yogurt, cheese). Animal protein sources contain all of the essential amino acids that your body needs to form its own various proteins.[1]

Plant-based diets, with no meat, eggs, or dairy, provide proteins mostly from legumes (beans, peas, lentils), nuts, seeds, grains (rice, wheat, corn, rye, oats, barley, quinoa), and vegetables. Although plant protein sources contain all of the essential amino acids in some quantity, each individual plant source can lack an *abundant* amount of one or more of the essential amino acids. Fortunately, the essential amino acids that are limited in one plant group may be easily obtained from another group that has higher quantities. For example, grains yield higher levels of certain essential amino acids while legumes supply higher levels of others. A balanced intake from a variety of plant sources can create a diet that contains a desirable level of all of the essential amino acids.[1]

Therefore, on a plant-based diet, it is important to consume a variety of plant-based protein sources, in quantities that will not only provide caloric energy but which, in combination, will supply proteins containing essential amino acids in amounts that are sufficient to maintain body protein homeostasis (stability at levels required to sustain normal functioning).[1,2] Complementing foods do not have to be eaten in the same meal. Rather, grains, legumes, soy products, nuts, seeds, and other vegetables can be eaten in variety over the course of the day to gain all of the necessary amino acids.[1,2]

The recipes and meal suggestions in this book are varied to provide rich sources of amino acids. Nutritional values have been calculated for each recipe, and the protein content is given for each serving. **Chapter 7** is dedicated to **Protein Matters**.

Nutrients of concern

It is important to include the nutrients calcium, vitamin D, vitamin B12, iodine, iron, zinc, choline, and omega-3 fatty acids in a healthy diet.[1-15] Deficiencies of these nutrients may result if they are not intentionally included, and this is especially true with a plant-based diet.

Detailed attention is paid to each individual nutrient of concern in **Chapter 8**. Strategies are provided to help ensure that the optimal levels of these nutrients are met. The stategies utilize natural food sources, fortified food sources, and dietary supplements as needed and in moderation. Understanding these strategies is important, as too much or too little of a particular nutrient may lead to harmful unintended consequences.[1]

Nutrient approximations for each recipe were made using multiple data sources including NutriBase 19 Pro+ Edition, v.19.1 (CyberSoft, Inc.), the United States Department of Agriculture (USDA), Agricultural Research Service Food Data Central, food labels, and from information supplied by manufacturers.

In summary:

- **Choose foods that will provide nutritional value. Eat enough nutrient-rich foods to provide energy, maintain a stable weight, and meet body protein requirements.**
- **Variety is essential. Be intentional about including a variety of plant protein sources in your meals.**
- **Ensure sufficient intake of nutrients of concern by utilizing natural food sources, fortified food sources, and dietary supplements as needed and in moderation (to bridge any nutrient gaps).**

Chapter 3: Meal Planning for a Plant-Based Diet

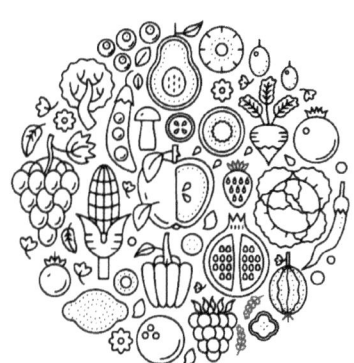

Choose menu items that will provide nutritional value

1. Recipes in the guide are accompanied by suggestions for easily prepared side items that can be included to complete a meal. In addition, permanent staples to consider as side items for any meal include:

    - Fresh fruits to add vitamins, fiber, and other phytonutrients.
    - Whole-grains (brown rice, whole-grain bread, whole-grain cereal) to help meet calorie and protein needs.
    - Plant milk fortified with calcium and protein to support bone health and supply amino acids.

    Side dishes can provide a diverse combination of required nutrients within the meal planning framework.

2. Personalize your meals further by adding protein from sources such as legumes (beans, peas, lentils), nuts, seeds, grains, vegetables, and plant-based protein shakes. Refer to **Chapter 7**, **Protein Matters**, for more on protein needs.

3. Attempt to fulfill your daily calorie and nutrient requirements within the framework of a scheduled meal pattern (breakfast, lunch, supper). Athletes and growing children/teens may benefit from a nutrient-dense snack in the mid-morning and mid-afternoon to help meet calorie and protein needs.[1-3] See **Chapter 5**, **Planning for Snacks and Desserts** to find more ideas about snacks.

Plan your menu and grocery list for the week

1. **Supper/Lunch/Breakfast**

   - Plan first for supper. Review the list of recipes and the sample menus in **Appendices A** and **B** for ideas. What looks good to eat this week?
   - Choose a main dish and side dish(es)/item(s) for each supper meal for the week. Plan to use leftovers or previously frozen meals on days when there will be little time to prepare a meal.
   - Write the names of the dishes and side items selected on your meal planning calendar.
   - Repeat the process for lunch and again for breakfast.

2. **Make a written grocery list that includes:**

   - Recipe ingredients needed for each meal (main and side dishes). Omit the ingredients you already have on hand.
   - Fruits for meals and snacks. Consider trying a new fruit that is in season. Make this part of the list flexible depending on what looks good in the store.
   - Beverages. Try plant milk that is fortified with vitamin B12, calcium, vitamin D, and protein. Refer to **Chapter 6**, **Beverages** for more on beverages.
   - Rice and/or bread as a side item to go with selected recipes.
   - Vegetables that are to be used as side items for the recipes you have chosen and have not already been added to your list. Include a few vegetables for lunch boxes and snacks. Ready-to-eat baby carrots, sugar snap peas, and broccoli florets are good choices. Make this part of the list flexible depending on what looks good in the store. Add a dressing for salads and a dip for vegetables to the list.

- Snacks for growing children/teens and athletes. Up to two snacks, a day should suffice (one snack mid-morning and one mid-afternoon as needed and desired). Refer to **Chapter 5**, **Planning for Snacks and Desserts** for snack ideas.
- Convenience items to keep in storage and prepare quickly. Bean and lentil soups, frozen plant-based chicken patties or burgers, and plant-based pizzas are examples. Keep some frozen vegetables on hand as well.
- Ingredients for any special dish or dessert that you plan to serve. See **Chapter 5**, **Planning for Snacks and Desserts** for more on special dessert ideas.

Making the recipes

1. Review your recipes the evening before making them. If dried beans are called for, begin soaking the beans so they are ready for use on the next day.

2. Identify a time to perform any other preparations that can be completed prior to cooking time to make the process go more quickly.

3. Freeze portions from recipes that make more than one or two meals to pull out later for quick meals. Portion enough for a family or individual meal into a container(s) with a label noting the contents and date.

What if I am eating out with friends and family?

1. Plant-based options at restaurants are becoming more common today. Looking at the menu online beforehand can be helpful to identify good options.

2. Offer to make a plant-based meal to share when staying with family and friends. You may interest others in plant-based eating by doing so.

3. When going on a trip or attending an event, consider eating plant-based foods beforehand. It can be helpful to keep a cooler handy for these occasions. If it is very difficult to keep your diet strictly plant-based, consider flexing to lacto-ovo vegetarian (includes dairy and eggs) or pesco-vegetarian (includes fish).

Chapter 4: Tips for Success

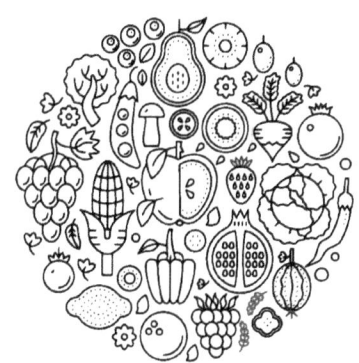

How to move the transitional process forward successfully

- **Be persistent.** Foods sometimes need to be offered many times before they are accepted. If someone doesn't like to eat a particular vegetable or fruit, especially in the case of a child, placing a small serving on their plate will make them more comfortable with that food. The more familiar a person is with a food, the more likely it is that they will choose that food either now or later in life, because tastes and preferences for foods evolve over time.[1,2]

- **Make hunger an asset.** Another way of presenting vegetables and fruits is to set one out before the meal is ready. Try using a less popular vegetable for an appetizer. As family members breeze through the kitchen, they may decide to try it! An avocado slice with a touch of salt might look a little tastier to a hungry individual when nothing else is offered.

- **Add some zest.** Adding a dressing on the side for raw vegetables may increase interest. Children in particular often like ranch dressing, and there are commercial plant-based ranch products available. Experiment with different dressings. Set several out at the same time in dipping bowls for variety and to improve familiarity.

- **Think small.** Cut fruits and vegetables into small pieces for young children for safety and to encourage acceptance. For example, peel a tangerine, break it into sections, remove any seeds, and cut the sections again into smaller pieces that can easily be picked up with fingers. When preparing a recipe, cut mushrooms or onions into tiny pieces (diced) so that a young child can more easily chew and swallow them. This method also gives the child a chance to gradually become accustomed to the flavors. Cutting a less popular vegetable into smaller pieces often improves acceptance by older children and adults as well.

- **Share the experience.** Sit down with your family for meals whenever possible. There is something special about sharing meals together. Simply seeing their parents eating the same foods that they are being served encourages children to eat and enjoy those foods.

- **Enlist little helpers.** Try to involve the whole family in the cooking process. Young children may enjoy helping to wash fruits and vegetables. As they grow older, they can also help to carefully measure ingredients. Getting children into the kitchen early gives them a valuable appreciation of the effort involved in preparing a meal.

- **Enlist bigger helpers.** Teach older children and teens to make the recipes in this book. Young adults who have mastered the recipes in this book will be armed with good nutrition principles to carry throughout their lives when they leave home. They will be able to prepare their own meals and share their good nutrition practices with their future families and friends to continue the cycle.

- **Let them choose.** Always try to give children a choice. When packing snacks and lunches ask which vegetable or fruit they would like: Carrot sticks or sugar snap peas? Apple slices or grapes? If they come home with uneaten food in their bag, wait until they finish their leftovers before offering another item they would prefer.

- **Grow it yourself.** Consider planting a garden or growing some potted herbs with your family. Having even a small garden with herbs and vegetables can be a memorable experience. When my children were very young, they would delightfully go around the garden picking and tasting the different herbs. Planting and pulling up vegetables like radishes is also fun. I still remember from my childhood the wonderful feeling of sitting in our garden and eating a fresh tomato off the vine or helping to pick turnip greens. My husband has fond memories of digging up potatoes when he was a child. This is another great way to increase familiarity and acceptance of vegetables. Safety note: it is a safe practice to wash herbs, fruits, and vegetables before eating them, even when they are organic, and it is important to teach children that some plants are poisonous.

- **May I have some more?** Adjust portion sizes for age and likeability. The serving size for an adult is not appropriate for a young child. Usually, the serving size for the very young (1-3 years) is about half of the adult serving size. For example, ¼ cup of rice, pasta, or cooked cereal is about one serving for a 1-year-old compared to ½ cup for an adult. Start out with smaller amounts for the very young, but allow them to eat as many servings as they wish. A plate with huge serving sizes may overwhelm a young child. Confidence levels will increase with serving sizes that are appropriate for age. Also, if the child doesn't really enjoy vegetables at all, giving them a smaller serving can be helpful. For example, giving a reticent 7-year-old just 4 sugar snap peas in their lunchbox as their vegetable serving instead of 8 will help them master eating vegetables and increase likeability.

- **Grain, grain that's the way.** Whole-grains supply nutrients such as vitamins and minerals and are often good sources of fiber which facilitates a cascade of beneficial health effects in the body. If early satiety from the fiber and bulk of a plant-based diet is a concern, as may be the case with some children who have small stomachs and big calorie needs, consider incorporating a few refined grains in meals as well. Additionally, more calories are absorbed from refined grains since they do not have the fiber and bulk of whole-grains.[3,4]

- **Be flexible.** Regularly or occasionally including some animal-based foods in a mostly plant-based diet may help long-term adherence and acceptance. Additional benefits from doing so include increased variety in meals and the opportunity to eat foods which contain nutrients that are less plentiful in a purely plant-based diet. However, following a plant-based diet more often than not will increase the likelihood of gaining the long-term health benefits associated with following a well-planned plant-based diet.

Chapter 5: Planning for Snacks and Desserts

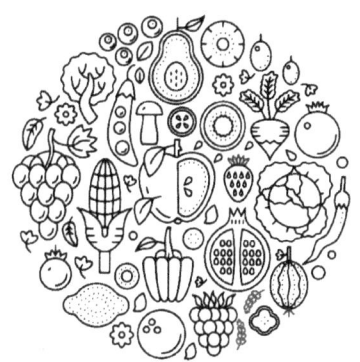

What about snacks?

For a growing and active child, teen, athlete, or someone trying to increase or maintain body mass, planned nutritious snacks can help meet calorie and protein needs. It is best to eat the snack around 2 hours before the next meal so that the meal time appetite will not be diminished. Also, if a child is not eating at meal times because they are full from their snack, consider making the snack smaller. Encourage water between meals in place of other beverages. Note that many of the snack items listed below may also be used as easily prepared complementary side dishes to provide additional nutrients for regular meals.

Snack ideas:

Apples, celery, or graham crackers with nut butter and raisins. Nut, seed, or bean butter are all good choices. Examples include sunflower seed butter, almond butter, soybean butter, or peanut butter. Try sunflower seed butter mixed with a little sweetener such as maple syrup or molasses.
Nut, seed, or bean butter on toast and plant milk containing protein (natural or fortified)

Popcorn, fruit (fresh or dried), and walnuts or almonds
Trail mix (consider: popcorn, pretzels, toasted oats O's or Cheerios® cereal, dried fruits, peanuts or toasted almond pieces, pumpkin seed kernels, sunflower seeds, coconut flakes, plant-based chocolate chips)
Pita bread slices or chips with hummus and grapes
Roasted chickpeas with olive oil and salt
Tortilla chips with salsa and beans or a burrito (beans, salsa, avocado, rice)
Frozen fruit and frozen soymilk (or any plant milk containing plant protein) made into a smoothie. Use ice cube trays to freeze the soymilk before adding everything to the blender.
Frozen chocolate or vanilla shake made from plant protein with or without fruit. Mix shake powder with a plant milk, freeze in ice cube trays, and then blenderize.
Raw vegetables and dressing on the side to dip (ex. sugar snap peas or carrots and plant-based ranch dressing) with a few crackers topped with nut, seed, or bean butter
Plant-based chicken sandwich or bean burger (divide into smaller serving sizes for children)

How to fit in desserts

Desserts can be a fun addition to a meal plan. However, for healthy habits and balanced meal planning purposes, limit desserts to a modest portion eaten one time a day or not at all depending on your family's preferences. Fresh fruit is really nature's most perfect dessert. Also, it is helpful to utilize convenience desserts over homemade desserts to allow the chef to focus energy on the more nutritious parts of the meal. If time allows for making desserts, there are two delicious recipes (Apple Crisp and Chocolate Chip Oatmeal Cookies) detailed in **The Recipes** section under **Desserts.**

Ideas for convenience plant-based desserts:

- Candied nuts
- Dried fruit pieces (blueberries, cherries, dates, sugared ginger pieces)

- Fig bars
- Frozen sorbet on a sugar or cake cone
- Frozen fruit bars
- Lemonade
- Plant-based chocolates (there are many, just turn over and read the labels)

Special care should be taken to reduce the risk of choking in a young child's diet or anyone who has chewing or swallowing difficulties.*

---

* The CDC has important information regarding potential choking hazards for young children. Please refer to their website https://ww.cdc.gov/ for more information.[1]

Chapter 6:
Beverages

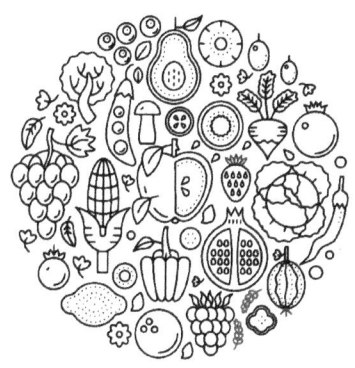

We need water

Drinking water throughout the day is a healthy habit to develop. Water is an important participant in biochemical reactions including filtering out wastes from our cells and delivering nutrients and oxygen to them.[1] It facilitates the movement of substances in our digestive and urinary tracts and is important in preventing constipation and bladder infections.[2,3] Another important reason to regularly drink water is to prevent the impairment of physical and mental abilities that may result from water deficiency.[4]

Filling up a water bottle at the beginning of the day can help improve overall intake by making access quick and easy. Because water is a significant component of most beverages, daily water needs can be met through beverages other than water. However, water is superior to sugary or alcoholic drinks since it is free of non-nutritious calories and additives such as artificial coloring and preservatives. Although beverages are the primary source, it is estimated that 20% of water requirements are usually gained through food consumption.[5]

On a plant-based diet, fluids/water intake should be regarded as:

1. a means of hydration (essential) and
2. as a vehicle which has the potential to incorporate and deliver additional protein, calcium, calories, and other nutrient requirements.

Tables 1 and 2 provide an example of daily beverage intake along with approximate adequate water intake guidelines.

Plant milk

On a plant-based diet, plant milk can help replace protein, calcium, and other nutrients found in animal-based products such as cow's milk. Plant milks are also lactose-free, which is helpful for persons who are intolerant of the milk sugar, lactose, found in animal-based milk. In nutrient content, soymilk is most similar to cow's milk. An 8-ounce cup of unsweetened soymilk contains about 80 calories, 4 grams of carbohydrate, and 7 grams of protein. It is often fortified with 300 to 450 milligrams of calcium.[6] Other plant milks (almond, cashew, coconut, flax, and hemp milk) require fortification to make them significant sources of protein and/or calcium. The protein fortification is often in the form of pea protein which increases calories and protein close to levels found in a cup of low-fat cow's milk.

While it is possible to find versions of plant milk that are protein-fortified, many of the varieties you may find at the market will not have this fortification. Without protein fortification and added sweeteners, plant milks (in particular almond, cashew, coconut, flax, and hemp milk) contain very little protein, or carbohydrate, and as little as 25 to 45 calories per cup.[6] This combination may be preferred for those watching carbohydrate or calorie content, especially if the plant milk offers calcium fortification.

Many plant milks are fortified with calcium and contain around 300-450 mg of that nutrient per 8-ounce cup. This can be a great help in meeting daily calcium needs for optimal bone health. In **Chapter 8**, **Nutrients of Concern**, the **Calcium** section contains a table showing the Recommended Dietary Allowances (RDAs) for calcium and a list of non-dairy foods (natural and fortified) in which calcium may be found.

What about juice?

Juice can be incorporated into a healthy diet in limited amounts. Over-consumption of juice may provide excess calories. The American Academy of Pediatrics recommends that children (ages 1-6) limit juice intake to ½-¾ cup (4-6 ounces) a day.[7] Juice, such as orange juice, can be found fortified with calcium which may assist in meeting total daily calcium needs. Small juice cups help with portion control. Also, it is better to eat the actual fruit or vegetable and gain the fiber and other phytonutrients that may be missing in juice alone. A fruit or vegetable smoothie is a good choice because it includes the entire edible fruit or vegetable. Smoothies can be added to meals or snacks. Since fruit smoothies contain concentrated sources of the natural sugar fructose, they may cause digestive upset in some susceptible persons, especially if consumed in large quantities.[4]

Table 1: Daily Beverage Intake (example for adult female)

Breakfast	1 cup tea or coffee and 1 cup plant milk such as unsweetened soymilk or other plant milk fortified with protein and calcium or ¾ cup orange juice fortified with calcium
Mid-morning	1 cup water
Lunch	1 cup plant milk such as unsweetened soymilk or other plant milk fortified with protein and calcium and 1 cup water
Mid-afternoon	1 cup water
Supper	1 cup plant milk such as unsweetened soymilk or other plant milk fortified with protein and calcium and 1 cup water
Evening	1 cup water

This example provides 2160 mL (9 cups) of fluid and about 900-1350 mg of calcium from beverages for the day. Note that males age 14 years and older and pregnant or lactating females (see Table 2) require 2-4 cups of water daily above the quantity provided in Table 1.

Table 2: Adequate Intakes* for Drinking Water (daily)

Recommendations include approximate water from all beverages and drinking water. About 20% of water comes from the food we eat which is not included in the table.

Age	Male	Female	Pregnancy	Lactation
0-6 months	3 cups**	3 cups**		
7-12 months	3 cups	3 cups		
1-3 years	4 cups	4 cups		
4-8 years	5 cups	5 cups		

9-13 years	8 cups	7 cups		
14-18 years	11 cups	8 cups	10 cups	13 cups
19-50 years	13 cups	9 cups	10 cups	13 cups
51-70 + years	13 cups	9 cups		

*Adequate Intake: This estimate is established when there is not enough evidence to give an RDA. This level is assumed to provide nutritional adequacy. It may be used as a general target for daily water intake in temperate climates by healthy adequately hydrated individuals with normal kidney function. Water needs will vary depending on medical conditions, medication intake, physical activity, and climates.
**This is assumed to be human breast milk.
1 liter (L) = 1,000 milliliters (mL) = approximately 4 cups. 240 mL = 1 cup
Source: 8

In summary:

- Drink plenty of water.
- Drink water throughout the day.
- Use fortified plant milk and small servings of fortified fruit juice to supplement dietary protein and/or calcium.

Chapter 7:
Protein Matters

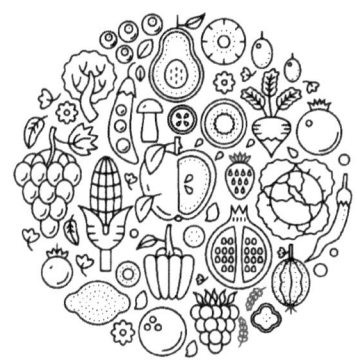

Consuming a variety of plant-based foods including grains, legumes, nuts, seeds, and other vegetables which collectively provide adequate amounts of calories and proteins helps to promote stability and normality in body functions.[1-3] As previously discussed in **Chapter 2**, meeting protein needs on a plant-based diet requires intentional planning. Recommended Dietary Allowances (RDAs) set by the Institute of Medicine, represent the average daily dietary intake levels for specific nutrients that meet the needs of nearly all (97 to 98 percent) healthy individuals within a particular group.[1]

Although no special adjustments to the RDA levels were recommended for vegetarians by the Institute of Medicine, other sources highlight the fact that not all plant protein is absorbed when eaten, because the protein is contained within the fibrous network of the plant and a considerable amount of fiber (with protein) leaves the body somewhat undigested.[1,4] They suggest that people following a strict plant-based diet should consume a greater amount of protein to make up for the reduced digestibility of some of the plant protein. Specifically, 1-1.1 grams protein/kilogram body weight/day (g/kg/d) was suggested for those adults versus the usual recommendation (RDA) of 0.8 g/kg/d.[1,4-8] This represents an increase of between 25-38% over the RDA.

In Table 1, the RDA suggested amounts of protein per day are given in the following form: grams of protein per kilogram of body weight per day (g/kg/d). Your weight in kg is equal to your weight in pounds (lb) divided by 2.2. For example, if you are an adult who weighs 120 lb, your weight in kg would be 54.5 kg. The RDA for protein in adults is 0.8 g/kg/d. Therefore, the RDA for protein for a 120 lb adult would be 54.5 kg times 0.8 g/kg/d, which rounds to about 44 g of protein per day. As mentioned above, it may be better for those following a strict plant-based diet to consume somewhat more.

Table 1: Recommended Dietary Allowances of Protein (Daily)

RDA (grams protein/kilogram body weight/day)

Age	Male	Female	Pregnancy*	Lactation
0-6 months**	1.52 g/kg/d	1.52 g/kg/d		
7-12 months	1.2 g/kg/d	1.2 g/kg/d		
1-3 years	1.05 g/kg/d	1.05 g/kg/d		
4-13 years	0.95 g/kg/d	0.95 g/kg/d		
14-18 years	0.85 g/kg/d	0.85 g/kg/d	1.1 g/kg/d	1.3 g/kg/d
19 + years	0.8 g/kg/d	0.8 g/kg/d	1.1 g/kg/d	1.3 g/kg/d

Note that some sources indicate an increase of 25-38% above the RDA is needed for those following a purely plant-based diet.
*Use pre-pregnancy weight for calculations.
**Adequate Intake: This estimate is established when there is not enough evidence to give an RDA. This level is assumed to provide nutritional adequacy.
Sources: 1,4-8

Special considerations for older adults and athletes

Because older adults (persons over 65 years of age) are less efficient at maintaining muscle mass and bone, some (but not all) research supports the inclusion of additional protein in the diet for this age group (1-1.2 g/kg/day of protein assuming normal kidney function).[7-11]

The Position of the Academy of Nutrition and Dietetics, Dietitians of Canada, and the American College of Sports Medicine: Nutrition and Athletic Performance suggest a total intake of 1.2-2.0 g/kg/day of protein for athletes to support normal body needs and additional performance requirements.[12]

Table 2: Selected Food Sources of Protein

Plant-Based Food Sources of Protein	
Beverages	
Almond milk, 1 cup (240 ml) fortified*	10 g
Flaxseed milk, 1 cup (240 ml) fortified*	8 g
Soymilk, 1 cup (240 ml)	8 g
Beans, Peas, Lentils	
Black beans, cooked, ½ cup (93 g)	8 g
Chickpeas, cooked, ½ cup (90 g)	7 g
Edamame, cooked, ½ cup (80 g)	9 g
Lentils, cooked, ½ cup (99 g)	9 g
Navy beans, cooked, ½ cup (91 g)	8 g
Seeds, Nuts	
Pumpkin seed kernels, dried, ¼ cup (32 g)	10 g
Almonds, whole, shelled, ¼ cup (36 g)	8 g
Walnuts, halves, ¼ cup (25 g)	4 g
Almond butter, 2 tablespoons (32 g)	7 g
Peanut butter, 2 tablespoons (32 g)	7-8 g
Sunflower seed butter, 2 tablespoons (32 g)	6 g

Soy Foods	
Tofu firm, ½ cup (126 g)	11 g
Tempeh, ½ cup (83 g)	17 g
Grains	
Amaranth, cooked, ½ cup (123 g)	5 g
Corn, cut, cooked, ½ cup (75 g)	3 g
Cream of wheat, cooked, 1 cup (244 g)	4 g
Oatmeal, cooked, 1 cup (240 g)	5 g
Pasta, durum wheat, 2 ounces (56 g)	8 g
Quinoa, cooked, ½ cup (93 g)	4 g
Rice, brown, cooked, ½ cup (98 g)	2 g
Vegetables	
Asparagus, cooked, ½ cup (90 g)	2 g
Broccoli, cooked, ½ cup (78 g)	2 g
Green peas, cooked, ½ cup (80 g)	4 g
Potato, baked, flesh and skin, 1 medium (173 g)	4 g
Potato, sweet, baked, flesh, 1 medium (151 g)	2 g
Spinach, cooked, ½ cup (90 g)	3 g
Turnip greens, cooked, ½ cup (82 g)	3 g

Animal-Based Food Sources of Protein	
Dairy, Eggs	
Milk, 1%, 1 cup (240 ml)	8 g
Greek yogurt, low-fat, 1 cup (227 g)	23 g
Mozzarella cheese, part-skim, 1 ounce (28 g)	7 g
Egg, 1 large (50 g)	6 g
Fish	
Herring, cooked, 3 ounces (85 g)	20 g
Salmon, sockeye, cooked, 3 ounces (85 g)	23 g
Sardines, canned in oil with bones, drained, 3 ounces (85 g)	21 g
Tuna, light, canned in water, drained, 3 ounces (85 g)	22 g

*Foods that have been fortified (nutrient added) with protein vary in the amount of fortification between food brands. Not all brands will be fortified.

ml = milliliters. g = grams.

Source: 13

In summary

- **Replacement of protein contained in animal-based food is an important consideration in selecting food for a plant-based diet. Intentionally including a variety of plant foods that are rich in protein and provide adequate calorie intake helps to assure protein replacement.**

- **Dietary protein may need to be increased to a level that is higher than the RDA for those persons following a purely plant-based diet, because some plant protein that is contained within the fibrous network of plants may not be fully digested and absorbed.**

- **Older adults and athletes may benefit by increasing their protein intake to levels above the RDA.**

Chapter 8: Nutrients of Concern and Summary Chart

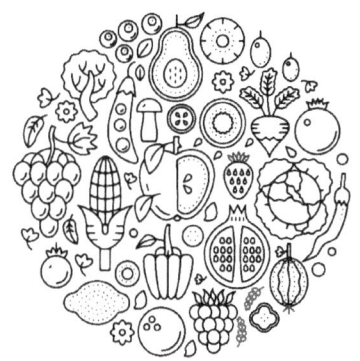

In this chapter, special attention will be directed toward certain nutrients that should be intentionally included in a plant-based diet, because obtaining them in adequate quantities may present a challenge. An understanding of this information is especially important for those who follow a purely plant-based diet. While specific attention may be required to gain these nutrients, it does not lessen the need to also provide sufficient calories, protein, and other nutrients to meet all recognized dietary adequacy standards. The nutrients of concern include: calcium, vitamin D, vitamin B12, iodine, iron, zinc, choline, and omega-3 fatty acids. Each nutrient page presents a widely accepted standard for the daily requirement of that nutrient (Recommended Dietary Allowance or Adequate Intake), and the nutrient's approximate amount per serving in certain foods. Strategies for meeting daily intake standards consider the nutrient's availability in natural and fortified foods, unique factors affecting absorption and retention in the body, and the use of nutrient supplements. While it is always best to meet nutritional requirements with natural or fortified whole food sources, if a shortfall remains between a nutrient requirement and an individual's intake of that nutrient from natural or fortified food, a nutrient supplement may be useful to bridge the nutrient gap.

Calcium

Calcium is an important mineral for a variety of health reasons including its support for strong bones.[1,2] Try to meet the Recommended Dietary Allowance (RDA) for calcium each day through your diet using natural and/or fortified sources such as some orange juice and plant milks. Most individuals should be able to meet their RDA for calcium by drinking 2-3 plant beverages that are fortified with calcium each day to augment the calcium in their natural food sources. Calcium is also found as a component of many multivitamins and in single supplement form. Adverse consequences may result from inadequate or excessive calcium intake. When calcium intake is the cause of excessive calcium levels in the body, the source of the excess is usually calcium supplements and not natural or calcium fortified food.[1]

Table 1: Recommended Dietary Allowances for Calcium (daily)

Age	Male	Female	Pregnancy/Lactation
0-6 months*	200 mg	200 mg	
7-12 months*	260 mg	260 mg	
1-3 years	700 mg	700 mg	
4-8 years	1,000 mg	1,000 mg	
9-13 years	1,300 mg	1,300 mg	
14-18 years	1,300 mg	1,300 mg	1,300 mg
19-50 years	1,000 mg	1,000 mg	1,000 mg
51-70 years	1,000 mg	1,200 mg	
71 + years	1,200 mg	1,200 mg	

*Adequate Intake: This estimate is established when there is not enough evidence to give an RDA. This level is assumed to provide nutritional adequacy.
mg = milligrams.
Source: 1

Table 2: Tolerable Upper Intake Levels* for Calcium (daily)

Age	Male/Female	Pregnancy/Lactation
0-6 months	1,000 mg	
7-12 months	1,500 mg	
1-8 years	2,500 mg	
9-18 years	3,000 mg	3,000 mg
19-50 years	2,500 mg	2,500 mg
51 + years	2,000 mg	

*Tolerable Upper Intake Level: The highest daily nutrient intake level that is not likely to cause unfavorable health effects.
mg = milligrams
Source: 1

Table 3: Selected Food Sources of Calcium

Plant-Based Food Sources of Calcium	
Beverages	
Almond milk, 1 cup (240 ml) fortified*	450 mg
Flaxseed milk, 1 cup (240 ml) fortified*	300 mg
Soymilk, 1 cup (240 ml) fortified*	300 mg
Orange juice, ¾ cup (180 ml) fortified*	261 mg
Beans, Peas, Lentils	
Chickpeas, cooked, ½ cup (90 g)	44 mg
Edamame, cooked, ½ cup (80 g)	49 mg

Great northern beans, cooked, ½ cup (90 g)	60 mg
Navy beans, cooked, ½ cup (91 g)	63 mg
Pinto beans, cooked, ½ cup (93 g)	40 mg
Seeds, Nuts	
Chia seeds, 1 tablespoon (11 g)	67 mg
Almonds, whole, shelled, ¼ cup (36 g)	96 mg
Brazil nuts, whole, shelled, ¼ cup (33 g)	53 mg
Soy Foods	
Tofu firm, prepared with calcium sulfate, ½ cup (126 g)**	253 mg
Grains	
Cream of wheat, cooked, 1 cup (244 g) fortified*	254 mg
Vegetables	
Broccoli, raw, 1 cup (91 g)	42 mg
Kale, cooked, ½ cup (59 g)	89 mg
Rhubarb, cooked with sugar, ½ cup (120 g)***	174 mg
Spinach, cooked, ½ cup (90 g)***	105 mg
Spinach, raw, 1 cup (30 g)***	30 mg
Turnip greens, cooked, ½ cup (73 g)	100 mg
Fruits	
Figs, dried, 3 (25 g)	41 mg
Prunes, dried, 3 (29 g)	12 mg

Other	
Blackstrap molasses, 1 tablespoon (15 ml)	100 mg
Animal-Based Food Sources of Calcium	
Dairy, Eggs	
Milk, 1%, 1 cup (240 ml)	300 mg
Greek yogurt, low-fat, 1 cup (227 g)	261 mg
Mozzarella cheese, part-skim, 1 ounce (28 g)	222 mg
Fish	
Salmon, pink, canned, with bones, 3 ounces (85 g)	241 mg
Salmon, pink, cooked, skinless, boneless, 3 ounces (85 g)	7 mg
Sardines, canned in oil with bones, drained, 3 ounces (85 g)	324 mg

*Foods that have been fortified (nutrient added) with calcium vary in the amount of fortification between food brands. Not all brands will be fortified.

**Tofu made with calcium salt. Tofu made without calcium salts contains little calcium.

***Oxalates are found in higher amounts in some vegetables such as spinach, beet greens, Swiss chard, and rhubarb. Oxalates may reduce calcium absorption.

ml = milliliters. g = grams. mg = milligrams.

Sources: 1,3

Vitamin D

Vitamin D supports calcium absorption, bone health, and immune function. Vitamin D can be obtained from exposure to sunlight, foods (natural and fortified sources), and supplements. Intake of too much or too little vitamin D has been linked with adverse health consequences. An excess of vitamin D usually comes from supplements and not from your diet or sunlight.[1]

From sunlight:

When ultraviolet sun rays reach the skin, vitamin D is produced. However, this process may be affected by many factors including time outdoors, sunscreen, clothing, time of year, distance from the equator, and skin pigmentation.[1] An assessment of your vitamin D level and plan for your individual needs that is based on your circumstances is best discussed with your healthcare provider.

From food:

Not many foods are naturally good sources of vitamin D. However, foods are increasingly being fortified with this vitamin. See Table 3 for selected plant-based food sources that are frequently fortified with vitamin D. Read food labels to help you assess your daily intake from foods.

From supplements:

Supplements may help meet daily vitamin D needs when factors such as time indoors, sunscreen, and food selection reduce your intake from natural sources. Vitamin D may be found in many multivitamins and as an individual supplement. Infants who are solely or partially breastfed may benefit from a vitamin D liquid drop supplement. It is a good idea to have vitamin D levels monitored periodically to ensure that those levels are within the ranges recommended for good health.

Table 1: Recommended Dietary Allowances for Vitamin D (daily)

Age	Male/Female	Pregnancy/Lactation
0-12 months*	10 mcg (400 IU)	
1-70 years	15 mcg (600 IU)	15 mcg (600 IU)
71 + years	20 mcg (800 IU)	

*Adequate Intake: This estimate is established when there is not enough evidence to give an RDA. This level is assumed to provide nutritional adequacy.
mcg = micrograms. IU = International Units. 40 IU = 1 mcg.
Source: 1

Table 2: Tolerable Upper Intake Levels* for Vitamin D (daily)

Age	Male/Female	Pregnancy/Lactation
0-6 months	25 mcg (1,000 IU)	
7-12 months	38 mcg (1,500 IU)	
1-3 years	63 mcg (2,500 IU)	
4-8 years	75 mcg (3,000 IU)	
9-19 + years	100 mcg (4,000 IU)	100 mcg (4,000 IU)

*Tolerable Upper Intake Level: The highest daily nutrient intake level that is not likely to cause unfavorable health effects.
mcg = micrograms. IU = International Units. 40 IU = 1 mcg
Source: 1

Table 3: Selected Food Sources of Vitamin D

Plant-Based Food Sources of Vitamin D	
Beverages	
Almond milk, 1 cup (240 ml) fortified*	2.5 mcg (101 IU)
Soymilk, 1 cup (240 ml) fortified*	3 mcg (120 IU)
Orange juice, ¾ cup (180 ml) fortified*	2 mcg (76 IU)
Fats	
Plant-based buttery spread, 1 tablespoon (14 g) fortified*	2 mcg (80 IU)
Smart Balance® Original Buttery Spread, 1 tablespoon (14 g) fortified*	4.2 mcg (168 IU)
Animal-Based Food Sources of Vitamin D	
Dairy, Eggs	
Milk, 1%, 1 cup (240 ml) fortified*	3 mcg (117 IU)
Egg, 1 large (50 g)	1 mcg (41 IU)
Fish	
Salmon, sockeye, cooked, 3 ounces (85 g)	14 mcg (560 IU)
Sardines, canned in oil with bones, drained, 3 ounces (85 g)	4 mcg (164 IU)
Cod liver oil, 1 tablespoon (15 ml)	34 mcg (1,360 IU)

*Foods that have been fortified (nutrient added) with vitamin D vary in the amount of fortification between food brands. Not all brands will be fortified. Check current food labels on products for the most up-to-date fortified amounts as product formulations may change over time.
ml = milliliters. g = grams. mcg = micrograms. IU = International Units. 40 IU = 1 mcg.
Source: 2

Vitamin B12

Vitamin B12 (cobalamin), a water-soluble vitamin, plays a critical role in the formation and functioning of our nervous system, blood cells, and DNA.[1-4] Symptoms of vitamin B12 deficiency may include fatigue, sore tongue, tingling in the hands and feet, dementia, osteoporosis, anemia, and cardiovascular disease. Significant developmental delays and neurological damage may be present in infants and toddlers who are deficient.

Vitamin B12 is found naturally in animal-based foods, rather than in plant-based foods. As a result, the group with a high risk for B12 deficiency includes vegetarians (not only those who follow a strict plant-based diet, but also those who consume milk and eggs). Moreover, pregnant or lactating vegetarian mothers and their infants, as well as persons with medical conditions that cause malabsorption problems (common in older adults) have an especially high risk of vitamin B12 deficiency.[2-4]

Fortunately, there are certain plant-based foods that are fortified with vitamin B12, including some cereals and various soymilks and other plant milks, which will have the fortification amounts reflected on their food labels. Oral supplements are another way to obtain this crucial vitamin.

Adequate intake of vitamin B12

Normally, the intrinsic factor (a protein made in the stomach), binds with vitamin B12 from food or supplements to enable absorption. Intrinsic factor can only bind with a small load of vitamin B12 at one time, so consuming a fortified food or a smaller dose vitamin B12 oral supplement a few times each day with several hours in between will help vitamin B12 absorption.[2,4,5] The Recommended Dietary Allowance (RDA) for vitamin B12 is currently set at 2.4 micrograms per day for adults (see Table 1 for the RDA for each age group). Some research suggests that amounts slightly higher than the RDAs are needed for optimal health.[6,7]

The body may also absorb a small percentage of ingested vitamin B12 through its passive diffusion mechanism, whereby the vitamin reaches the blood by diffusing through the intestinal wall.[5] Because only a small percentage of available vitamin B12 is absorbed by this mechanism, higher dose oral supplements can also be used to maximize the opportunity for the passive diffusion process to help meet vitamin B12 needs.[2,3,8] Vitamin B12 supplements are available in multivitamin and single vitamin tablets. These products frequently contain an amount of vitamin B12 that is much greater than the RDA, because of the low absorption potential of vitamin B12 taken all at once.

To ensure adequate intake, vegetarians may consider one or both of the strategies listed above to meet their requirements for this very important vitamin. Follow the advice of your personal qualified healthcare provider to adopt the protocol for maintaining vitamin B12 that is best for your specific needs. The vitamin B12 level in vegetarians and others at risk for deficiency should be checked periodically by your healthcare provider. [3,8]

Table 1: Recommended Dietary Allowances for Vitamin B12 (daily)

Age	Male/Female	Pregnancy	Lactation
0-6 months*	0.4 mcg		
7-12 months*	0.5 mcg		
1-3 years	0.9 mcg		
4-8 years	1.2 mcg		
9-13 years	1.8 mcg		
14 + years	2.4 mcg	2.6 mcg	2.8 mcg

*Adequate Intake: This estimate is established when there is not enough evidence to give an RDA. This level is assumed to provide nutritional adequacy.

mcg = micrograms.

Source: 1

Table 2: Selected Food Sources of Vitamin B12

Plant-Based Food Sources of Vitamin B12	
Beverages	
Almond milk, 1 cup (240 ml) fortified*	3 mcg
Soymilk, 1 cup (240 ml) fortified*	2.7 mcg
Grains	
Raisin bran cereal, 1 cup (59 g) fortified*	1.4 mcg
Total® cereal, 1 cup (40 g) fortified*	2 mcg
Other	
Nutritional yeast, 1 tablespoon (9 g) fortified*	14 mcg
Animal-Based Food Sources of Vitamin B12	
Dairy, Eggs	
Milk, 1%, 1 cup (240 ml)	1 mcg
Greek yogurt, low-fat, 1 cup (227 g)	1.2 mcg
Egg, 1 large (50 g)	0.4 mcg
Fish	
Salmon, sockeye, cooked, 3 ounces (85 g)	3.8 mcg

*Foods that have been fortified (nutrient added) with vitamin B12 vary in the amount of fortification between food brands. Not all brands will be fortified. Check current food labels on products for the most up-to-date fortified amounts as product formulations may change over time.

ml = milliliters. g = grams. mcg = micrograms.

Source: 9

Iodine

Iodine is a trace element that plays an important role in the formation of thyroid hormones. These hormones are essential for regulating metabolism and normal growth and development. Iodine is available in foods (natural and fortified sources) and supplements (multivitamin and single). Too much or too little iodine can be harmful to health.[1]

Food sources of iodine vary, depending on the particular food and the iodine content in the soil where the food was grown. Seafood (seaweed and saltwater fish), dairy products, and iodized salt are common sources of iodine. Because some of the common foods containing iodine are not part of a plant-based diet, those following this diet must pay special attention to their daily intake of iodine.

To help meet the nutrient requirements for iodine, use a food product that is fortified with a known amount of iodine, such as iodized salt when called for in recipes and for mealtime seasoning, but take care to use salt moderately and follow any salt use restrictions from your health care provider. If you are unable to meet the daily Recommended Dietary Allowance (RDA) for your age through food alone, consider a routine iodine supplement to bridge your nutrient gap.

Table 1: Recommended Dietary Allowances for Iodine (daily)

Age	Male/Female	Pregnancy	Lactation
0-6 months	110 mcg*		
7-12 months	130 mcg*		
1-8 years	90 mcg		
9-13 years	120 mcg		
14-19 + years	150 mcg	220 mcg	290 mcg

*Adequate Intake: This estimate is established when there is not enough evidence to give an RDA. This level is assumed to provide nutritional adequacy.

mcg = micrograms.

Source: 1

Table 2: Tolerable Upper Intake Levels* for Iodine (daily)

Age	Male/Female	Pregnancy/Lactation
0-12 months	Not available—obtain through breast milk, formula, and food	
1-3 years	200 mcg	
4-8 years	300 mcg	
9-13 years	600 mcg	
14-18 years	900 mcg	900 mcg
19 + years	1,100 mcg	1,100 mcg

*Tolerable Upper Intake Level: The highest daily nutrient intake level that is not likely to cause unfavorable health effects.

mcg = micrograms.

Source: 1

Table 3: Selected Food Sources of Iodine

Plant-Based Food Sources of Iodine	
Vegetable	
Seaweed, nori, 1 sheet (2.5 g)*	35 mcg
Seasoning	
Iodized table salt, ¼ teaspoon (1.5 g) fortified**	78 mcg
Animal-Based Food Sources of Iodine	
Dairy, Eggs	
Milk, 1%, 1 cup (240 ml)	89 mcg

Greek yogurt, non-fat, 1 cup (227 g)	116 mcg
Egg, 1 large (50 g)	25 mcg
Fish	
Cod, baked, 3 ounces (85 g)	158 mcg
Salmon, sockeye, canned, drained, 3 ounces (85 g)	13 mcg
Shrimp, cooked, 3 ounces (85 g)	13 mcg
Tuna, light, canned in water, drained, 3 ounces (85 g)	7 mcg

*Iodine content in seaweed varies widely, and some contain large amounts. Therefore, it is not advisable to consume large quantities of seaweed due to the risk of iodine toxicity.

**Foods that have been fortified (nutrient added) with iodine vary in the amount of fortification between food brands. Not all brands will be fortified.

ml = milliliters. g = grams. mcg = micrograms.

Sources: 1,2

Iron

Iron is an essential mineral that is crucial for growth and development, oxygen metabolism, and many other important functions. Iron is found in hemoglobin, a red blood cell protein that carries oxygen from the lungs to tissues throughout the body. It is also found in myoglobin, a muscle tissue protein that delivers oxygen to muscle cells.[1] Deficiency in iron can negatively affect cognitive development, immune system functioning, and temperature regulation. Fatigue, rapid heartbeat and palpitations are some possible deficiency symptoms.[1]

While many plant foods (natural and fortified) are rich sources of iron (Table 3), dietary components such as phytates and polyphenols may reduce iron absorption.[2,3] However, consuming vitamin C-rich foods along with iron sources enhances the absorption of iron.[1,2] Some foods high in vitamin C include oranges, grapefruit, lemons and limes, strawberries, kiwi, tomatoes, broccoli, bell peppers, and kale. Screening for iron status periodically, including serum ferritin, is prudent while following a predominantly plant-based diet.[1,4]

Young children as well as pregnant and menstruating women are at a higher risk for iron deficiency.[1] Vegetarian athletes who regularly perform at intense levels are also at risk for deficiency, and it has been suggested that athletes may need as much as 70% more iron than the Recommended Dietary Allowances (RDAs).[5,6]

To meet the recommended daily nutritional needs for iron (RDA), pay attention to the amounts taken in daily from foods (natural and fortified) by checking food content references and reading nutrition labels. Most individuals who are not at elevated risk for iron deficiency should be able to meet their RDA for iron by carefully selecting natural and fortified sources of iron for their meals. Low-dose iron supplements, under the direction of a physician, are a reasonable consideration for persons who are at greater risk for deficiency because of their higher RDA or circumstantial requirements and for others who are not meeting their needs with natural and fortified foods within their diet. Supplemental iron is available in many multivitamins and as a single supplement. However, too much iron can contribute to cellular damage which may lead to numerous chronic disease conditions including organ failure, vascular diseases, diabetes, and others.[5,7-9] Avoid excessive supplementation. Also, note that accidental overdose of iron-containing products is a leading cause of fatal poisoning in children under 6. Keep this product out of reach of children. Call a poison control center or doctor immediately if an accidental overdose occurs.[1]

Table 1: Recommended Dietary Allowances for Iron (daily)

Age	Male	Female	Pregnancy	Lactation
0-6 months	0.27 mg*	0.27 mg*		
7-12 months	11 mg	11 mg		
1-3 years	7 mg	7 mg		
4-8 years	10 mg	10 mg		
9-13 years	8 mg	8 mg		
14-18 years	11 mg	15 mg	27 mg	10 mg
19-50 years	8 mg	18 mg	27 mg	9 mg
51+ years	8 mg	8 mg		

*Adequate Intake: This is based on healthy infants' average consumption of iron through breast milk. This estimate is established when there is not enough evidence to give an RDA and is assumed to provide nutritional adequacy. For full-term infants between 4-6 months of age, complementary iron-fortified cereals may be started as well as other iron-rich foods in a consistency appropriate for age and development. Iron supplementation may also be recommended by your physician. Iron-fortified formulas are suggested for infants not consuming breast milk.

mg = milligrams.
Sources: 1,2,10,11

Table 2: Tolerable Upper Intake Levels* for Iron (daily)

Age	Male/Female	Pregnancy/Lactation
0-13 years	40 mg	
14 + years	45 mg	45 mg

*Tolerable Upper Intake Level: The highest daily nutrient intake level that is not likely to cause unfavorable health effects.
mg = milligrams.
Source: 1

Table 3: Selected Food Sources of Iron

Plant-Based Food Sources of Iron	
Beverages	
Soymilk, 1 cup (240 ml)	1-1.5 mg
Beans, Peas, Lentils	
Black-eyed peas, cooked, ½ cup (93 g)	2 mg
Chickpeas, cooked, ½ cup (90 g)	2.6 mg
Edamame, cooked, ½ cup (78 g)	1.8 mg
Kidney beans, cooked, ½ cup (89 g)	2.6 mg
Lentils, cooked, ½ cup (99 g)	3.3 mg
White beans, cooked, ½ cup (90 g)	3.3 mg
Seeds, Nuts	
Pumpkin seed kernels, dried, ¼ cup (32 g)	2.8 mg
Almonds, whole, shelled, ¼ cup (36 g)	1.3 mg

Almond butter, 2 tablespoons (32 g)	1.1 mg
Peanut butter, 2 tablespoons (32 g)	0.6 mg
Sunflower seed butter, 2 tablespoons (32 g)	1.3 mg
Soy Foods	
Tofu, firm, ½ cup (126 g)	3.4 mg
Grains	
Cream of wheat, cooked, 1 cup (244 g) fortified*	10 mg
Oatmeal, cooked, 1 cup (240 g)	1.6 mg
Quinoa, cooked, ½ cup (93 g)	1.4 mg
Rice, brown, cooked, ½ cup (98 g)	0.5 mg
Cheerios® cereal, 1 cup (26 g) fortified*	8.4 mg
Grape-Nuts® cereal, ½ cup (58 g) fortified*	16.2 mg
Raisin Bran cereal, 1 cup (59 g) fortified*	8-11 mg
Total® cereal, 1 cup (40 g) fortified*	18 mg
Vegetables	
Baked potato, flesh and skin, 1 medium (173 g)	1.9 mg
Broccoli, boiled, ½ cup (92 g)	0.6 mg
Spinach, boiled, ½ cup (90 g)	3.2 mg
Tomatoes, stewed, ½ cup (51 g)	1 mg
Fruits	
Raisins, ¼ cup (41 g)	1 mg

Other	
Dark chocolate (45-59% cacao solids), 1 ounce (28 g)	2.3 mg
Molasses, 2 tablespoons (40 g)	1.9 mg
Animal-Based Food Sources of Iron	
Eggs	
Egg, 1 large (50 g)	1 mg
Fish	
Tuna, light, canned in water, drained, 3 ounces (85 g)	1.3 mg

*Foods that have been fortified (nutrient added) with iron vary in the amount of fortification between food brands. Not all brands will be fortified. Check current food labels on products for the most up-to-date fortified amounts as product formulations may change over time.
ml = milliliters. g = grams. mg = milligrams.
Source: 12

Zinc

Zinc is an essential mineral that is important for growth, sexual development, proper immune system functioning, skin integrity, and taste and smell. Good plant-based food sources for zinc include whole-grains, legumes, nuts, and seeds. Many breakfast cereals are also fortified with zinc.[1]

Available levels of zinc from plant-based food sources are generally lower than those from animal-based sources. Phytates are plant components that bind with zinc and reduce zinc absorption. Phytates are found in higher amounts in whole-grains, legumes, nuts, and seeds.[1] There are a number of cooking or processing methods that will reduce phytates. A few examples are soaking beans, sprouting beans, and leavening bread, especially by using yeast. Allowing ample time for the bread to rise and break down phytates improves zinc absorption.[1-5] Some lentils and beans may be bought already sprouted. Although they reduce zinc absorption, phytates have good qualities as well, as they are strong antioxidants, and may reduce the risk of cancer and other chronic diseases.[2,4,6]

It is important to consume the recommended amounts of zinc (Recommended Dietary Allowance-RDA) consistently. The RDAs for zinc, shown in Table 1, should be met daily because the body does not have a good storage system for this mineral.[1] Note that during pregnancy and breastfeeding, zinc recommendations are higher than at other times. Some signs of a possible zinc deficiency include slowed growth for children, loss of appetite, and impaired immunity which should be quickly assessed by your qualified healthcare provider.[7]

Breastfed infants should receive an adequate intake of 2 milligrams (mg) of zinc for the first 4-6 months but will need daily zinc sources from foods, fortified foods, and possibly supplements to meet recommended needs thereafter, with care taken not to exceed the Tolerable Upper Intake Level (Table 2).[1] Many infant cereals are fortified with zinc. Zinc is also commonly added to multivitamin supplements.

Table 1: Recommended Dietary Allowances for Zinc (daily)

Age	Male	Female	Pregnancy	Lactation
0-6 months	2 mg*	2 mg*		
7-12 months	3 mg	3 mg		

Age				
1-3 years	3 mg	3 mg		
4-8 years	5 mg	5 mg		
9-13 years	8 mg	8 mg		
14-18 years	11 mg	9 mg	12 mg	13 mg
19+ years	11 mg	8 mg	11 mg	12 mg

*Adequate Intake: This estimate is established when there is not enough evidence to give an RDA. This level is assumed to provide nutritional adequacy.
mg = milligrams.
Source: 8

Table 2: Tolerable Upper Intake Levels* for Zinc (daily)

Age	Male/Female	Pregnancy/Lactation
0-6 months	4 mg	
7-12 months	5 mg	
1-3 years	7 mg	
4-8 years	12 mg	
9-13 years	23 mg	
14-18 years	34 mg	34 mg
19+ years	40 mg	40 mg

*Tolerable Upper Intake Level: The highest daily nutrient intake level that is not likely to cause unfavorable health effects.
mg = milligrams.
Source: 8

Table 3: Selected Food Sources of Zinc

Plant-Based Food Sources of Zinc	
Beverages	
Soymilk, 1 cup (240 ml)	0.6 mg
Beans, Peas, Lentils	
Black beans, cooked, ½ cup (93 g)	0.7 mg
Black-eyed peas, cooked, ½ cup (86 g)	1.1 mg
Chickpeas, cooked, ½ cup (82 g)	1.3 mg
Edamame, cooked, ½ cup (78 g)	1.1 mg
Kidney beans, cooked, ½ cup (89 g)	0.9 mg
Lentils, cooked, ½ cup (99 g)	1.3 mg
Lima beans, cooked, ½ cup (94 g)	0.9 mg
Navy beans, cooked, ½ cup (91 g)	0.9 mg
Split peas, cooked, ½ cup (98 g)	1 mg
Seeds, Nuts	
Pumpkin seed kernels, ¼ cup (32 g)	2.5 mg
Sesame seeds, dried, 1 tablespoon (9 g)	0.7 mg
Sunflower seed kernels, 2 tablespoons (18 g)	1 mg
Almonds, whole, shelled, ¼ cup (36 g)	1.1 mg
Cashews, halves and whole, ¼ cup (34 g)	1.9 mg
Pecans, ¼ cup (27 g)	1.2 mg

Walnuts, halves, ¼ cup (25 g)	0.8 mg
Cashew butter, 2 tablespoons (32 g)	1.7 mg
Peanut butter, 2 tablespoons (32 g)	0.8-0.9 mg
Sunflower seed butter, 2 tablespoons (32 g)	1.6 mg
Soy Foods	
Tempeh, ½ cup (83 g)	0.9 mg
Tofu, firm, raw, ½ cup (126 g)	2 mg
Grains	
Oatmeal, cooked, 1 cup (240 g)	1.5 mg
Quinoa, cooked, ½ cup (93 g)	1 mg
Rice, brown, cooked, ½ cup (99 g)	0.7 mg
Rice, wild, cooked, ½ cup (82 g)	1.1 mg
Whole wheat bread, 1 ounce, 1 slice (32 g)	0.6 mg
Cheerios® cereal, 1 cup (26 g) fortified*	1.5 mg
Grape-Nuts® cereal, ½ cup (58 g) fortified*	3.3 mg
Raisin Bran cereal, 1 cup (59 g) fortified*	2-15 mg
Total® cereal, 1 cup (40 g) fortified*	11 mg
Vegetables	
Asparagus, cooked, ½ cup (90 g)	0.5 mg
Avocados, pureed, ½ cup (115 g)	0.8 mg
Green peas, cooked, ½ cup (80 g)	1 mg

Mushrooms, white, cooked, ½ cup (78 g)	0.7 mg
Spinach, cooked, ½ cup (90 g)	0.7 mg
Other	
Nutritional yeast, 1 tablespoon (5 g)	1 mg
Animal-Based Food Sources of Zinc	
Dairy, Eggs	
Milk, 1%, 1 cup (240 ml)	1 mg
Greek yogurt, low-fat, 1 cup (227 g)	1.4 mg
Egg, 1 large (50 g)	0.6 mg
Fish	
Salmon, sockeye, cooked, 3 ounces (85 g)	0.5 mg

*Foods that have been fortified (nutrient added) with zinc vary in the amount of fortification between food brands. Not all brands will be fortified. Check current food labels on products for the most up-to-date fortified amounts as product formulations may change over time.
ml = milliliters. g = grams. mg = milligrams.
Source: 9

Choline

Choline is a critical nutrient involved in the formation and composition of cell membranes. It plays a role in numerous nervous system activities such as memory, muscle control, and early brain development. It is also necessary for proper liver function.[1,2]

Part of the body's choline requirement is produced in the liver. The remaining amount, estimated by the Adequate Intake (Table 1), comes from the diet. Choline can be found in a wide range of foods and also as supplements. Many of the foods highest in choline come from animal sources. Therefore, anyone following a plant-based diet may be at risk for choline insufficiency. While it is best to gain nutrients primarily through foods, supplements may help make up for any deficits. As with other vitamins and minerals, excessive supplementation may have negative effects.[1,2]

Table 1: Adequate Intakes* for Choline (daily)

Age	Male	Female	Pregnancy	Lactation
0-6 months	125 mg	125 mg		
7-12 months	150 mg	150 mg		
1-3 years	200 mg	200 mg		
4-8 years	250 mg	250 mg		
9-13 years	375 mg	375 mg		
14-18 years	550 mg	400 mg	450 mg	550 mg
19+ years	550 mg	425 mg	450 mg	550 mg

*Adequate Intake: This estimate is established when there is not enough evidence to give an RDA. This level is assumed to provide nutritional adequacy.
mg = milligrams.
Source: 1

Table 2: Tolerable Upper Intake Levels* for Choline (daily)

Age	Male/Female	Pregnancy/Lactation
0-12 months	Not available—obtain through breast milk, formula, and food	
1-8 years	1,000 mg	
9-13 years	2,000 mg	
14-18 years	3,000 mg	3,000 mg
19+ years	3,500 mg	3,500 mg

*Tolerable Upper Intake Level: The highest daily nutrient intake level that is not likely to cause unfavorable health effects.

mg = milligrams.

Source: 1

Table 3: Selected Food Sources of Choline

Plant-Based Food Sources of Choline	
Beverages	
Soymilk, 1 cup (240 ml)	57 mg
Beans, Peas, Lentils	
Chickpeas, cooked, ½ cup (90 g)	38 mg
Edamame, cooked, ½ cup (80 g)	44 mg
Kidney beans, cooked, ½ cup (89 g)	27 mg
Pinto beans, cooked, ½ cup (86 g)	30 mg
Split peas, cooked, ½ cup (80 g)	30 mg

Seeds, Nuts	
Sunflower seed kernels, 2 tablespoons (18 g)	10 mg
Almonds, whole, shelled, ¼ cup (36 g)	19 mg
Peanuts, ¼ cup (37 g)	24 mg
Peanut butter, 2 tablespoons (32 g)	20 mg
Soy Foods	
Tofu, firm, ½ cup (126 g)	35 mg
Grains	
Quinoa, cooked, ½ cup (93 g)	22 mg
Wheat germ, 1 tablespoon (7 g)	13 mg
Vegetables	
Asparagus, cooked, ½ cup (90 g)	24 mg
Broccoli, cooked, ½ cup (78 g)	31 mg
Brussels sprouts, cooked, ½ cup (78 g)	32 mg
Cauliflower, cooked, ½ cup (62 g)	24 mg
Green peas, cooked, ½ cup (80 g)	24 mg
Red potato, baked, flesh and skin, 1 large (299 g)	57 mg
Animal-Based Food Sources of Choline	
Dairy, Eggs	
Milk, 1% fat, 1 cup (240 ml)	43 mg
Greek yogurt, low-fat, 1 cup (227 g)	35 mg

Egg, 1 large (50 g)	169 mg
Fish	
Atlantic Cod, cooked, 3 ounces (85 g)	71 mg
Salmon, sockeye, cooked, 3 ounces (85 g)	96 mg

ml = milliliters. g = grams. mg = milligrams.
Sources: 1,3

Omega 3 Fatty Acids

Alpha-linolenic acid (ALA) from the omega-3 fatty acid family is an essential fatty acid. ALA is easily acquired through a plant-based diet because it is found in plentiful amounts in nuts and seeds including walnuts, flaxseeds, chia seeds, hemp seeds, and plant oils (flaxseed, canola, and soybean).[1]

Current research findings indicate that, in addition to the essential fatty acid ALA, there is evidence of beneficial effects from two other omega-3 fatty acids, eicosapentaenoic acid (EPA) and docosahexaenoic acid (DHA). EPA and DHA have been associated with decreasing inflammation in the body, and offering protective effects for the cardiovascular system.[1-3] DHA is also present in high amounts in tissues in the brain, eyes, and sperm, and some studies have shown it may positively affect cognitive functioning at different times in the life cycle.[1-5]

The body can convert ALA into DHA and EPA in limited amounts. Even with this conversion of the plentiful supply of ALA found in plant-based foods, blood levels of EPA and DHA in vegetarians are generally lower than in non-vegetarians.[6]

On a purely plant-based diet, suggestions for promoting a desirable profile of omega-3 fatty acids in the body include increasing the intake of ALA by 2 grams per day to increase the body's conversion rate of ALA to EPA and DHA.[2,6,7] For reference, 1 teaspoon of flaxseed oil provides 2.4 grams of ALA.[2] Alternatively, taking low-dose (200-300 mg per day) plant-based microalgae EPA and DHA supplements can also increase EPA and DHA in the body.[2,6,8] Microalgae is the original plant source that fish consume to acquire those fatty acids.[1]

Non-plant-based food sources of EPA and DHA include certain fatty fish and seafood (herring, salmon, sardines, trout, and tuna*).[1] Other food products which are fortified with these fatty acids are also becoming increasingly available.

As with other nutrients, too much may have harmful effects. Consult your qualified healthcare professional before significantly increasing your intake.

Table 1: Adequate Intakes* for ALA (daily)

---

* The FDA has issued advice regarding eating fish. Refer to its website, https://www.fda.gov for the latest guidelines.[9]

Age	Male	Female	Pregnancy	Lactation
0-12 months**	0.5 g	0.5 g		
1-3 years	0.7 g	0.7 g		
4-8 years	0.9 g	0.9 g		
9-13 years	1.2 g	1 g		
14+ years	1.6 g	1.1 g	1.4 g	1.3 g

*Adequate Intake: This estimate is established when there is not enough evidence to give an RDA. This level is assumed to provide nutritional adequacy.
**As total omega-3s. All other values are for ALA alone. Omega-3s come through breast milk or through formulas with at least 500 mg omega-3s for non-breastfeeding infants.
g = grams.
Source: 1

Table 2: Selected Food Sources of ALA, EPA, DHA

Plant-Based Food Sources of Omega-3s	ALA	EPA	DHA
Beverages			
Soymilk, 1 cup (240 ml)	0.4 g		
Beans			
Edamame, cooked, ½ cup (78 g)	0.28 g		
Seeds, Nuts			
Chia seeds, 1 tablespoon (11 g)	1.9 g		
Flaxseeds, 1 tablespoon (11 g)	2.39 g		
Hemp seeds, 1 tablespoon (10 g)	0.87 g		
Walnuts, halves, ¼ cup (25 g)	2.27 g		

Fats, Oils			
Canola oil, 1 tablespoon (15 ml)	1.28 g		
Flaxseed oil, cold-pressed, 1 tablespoon (15 ml)	7.26 g		
Soybean oil, 1 tablespoon (15 ml)	0.92 g		
Earth Balance® Vegan Buttery Sticks, 1 tablespoon (14 g)*	0.32 g		
Smart Balance® Original Buttery Spread, 1 tablespoon (14 g)*	0.4 g		
Animal-Based Food Sources of Omega-3s			
Dairy, Eggs			
Milk, 1% fat, 1 cup (240 ml)	0.01 g		
Egg, 1 large (50 g)	0.02 g		0.03 g
Fish			
Herring, cooked, 3 ounces (85 g)		0.76 g	0.92 g
Salmon, sockeye, cooked, 3 ounces (85 g)	0.05 g	0.25 g	0.48 g
Sardines, canned in oil with bones, drained 3 ounces (85 g)		0.4 g	0.43 g
Trout, rainbow, wild, cooked, 3 ounces (85 g)		0.4 g	0.44 g
Tuna, light, canned in water, drained, 3 ounces (85 g)		0.04 g	0.19 g

*Check current food labels on products for the most up-to-date amounts as product formulations may change over time.

ml = milliliters. g = grams. To convert from grams to milligrams multiply the number of grams by 1,000. Example: Herring 3 ounces = 0.92 g DHA X 1,000 = 920 mg DHA.

Sources: 1,10

Nutrients of Concern: Summary Chart*

Calcium: Consume natural and fortified sources of high calcium foods daily to meet the RDA. Consider including 2-3 calcium-fortified beverages daily.
Vitamin D: Include foods fortified in vitamin D. Consider a vitamin D supplement daily to meet the RDA for age, especially if wearing daily sunscreen or staying indoors much of the day.
Vitamin B12: Include reliable fortified food sources of vitamin B12 and/or smaller dose supplements daily to meet your needs. Consider taking larger dose vitamin B12 supplements a few times a week for additional support. Follow the advice of your qualified healthcare provider as to the best vitamin B12 protocol for your specific needs. Check your vitamin B12 level periodically.
Iodine: Use fortified foods containing known amounts such as iodized salt when called for in recipes and/or flavoring to help ensure recommended requirements (RDA). Consider taking an iodine supplement regularly to bridge any remaining nutrient gaps to meet the RDA for your age.
Iron: Pay attention to daily iron intake. Include natural and fortified foods (example: iron fortified dry ready-to-eat cereal) to meet daily needs (RDA). Fruits and other vitamin C sources will enhance iron absorption. If needs are not being met with foods (natural and fortified), consider a low-dose iron supplement to bridge gaps under the care of a physician. Consider routine lab monitoring if at risk for deficiency and periodic screening, if concerned, for all persons. Avoid excessive supplementation. Secure supplements away from young children.
Zinc: Include foods that are natural and fortified sources of zinc daily (example: zinc fortified dry ready-to-eat cereal). Meet RDA levels with daily consistency. If needs are not being met with foods alone, a low-dose zinc supplement can help bridge the nutrient gap for optimal intake.
Choline: Include food sources of choline daily. If Adequate Intake recommended levels are not being met with foods, consider taking a choline supplement to bridge the gap.
Omega-3 fatty acids: Increase intake of foods with high ALA content, and consider including a small dose of algal oil DHA and EPA supplement daily to support a more desirable omega-3 fatty acid profile in the body.

*These suggestions are meant to highlight information about certain nutrients that may be of concern for healthy persons following a predominantly plant-based diet. They are not meant to take the place of medical advice from your physician.

Supplements

Obtaining most of your nutrients through natural or fortified foods is desirable when possible. However, supplements can also be utilized to supply nutrient support for nutritional needs that are not being met by food alone.

Supplements are available for many nutrients and may be plant-based or animal-based. Supplements may contain single or multiple nutrients in varying amounts. Often, a multivitamin will contain several of the previously mentioned nutrients of concern, as well as a number of additional substances (primarily vitamins and minerals) required by your body. As each multivitamin is different, read the labels to find the one that best meets your needs. Other nutritional supplements may be consumed individually when necessary to provide additional calories, protein, or specific nutrients. Nutritional supplements come in many forms (liquid, chewable, dissolvable, or pill) to accommodate swallowing abilities. Sometimes, adding a little maple syrup or tart juice to a poor-tasting supplement can make it more palatable. Keep in mind that some supplements may need to be taken with food to enable absorption or prevent nausea. To ensure the safe application of supplements to your diet, discuss your dietary intake, supplement use, and concerns with your doctor and registered dietitian nutritionist so that an assessment and plan for your individual needs can be made.

All supplements should be kept out of reach of children. The Food and Drug Administration requires iron-containing products to carry a label that states, "Accidental overdose of iron-containing products are a leading cause of fatal poisoning in children under 6. Keep this product out of reach of children. In case of accidental overdose, call a doctor or poison control center immediately."

Part 2:
Cooking Essentials and Recipes

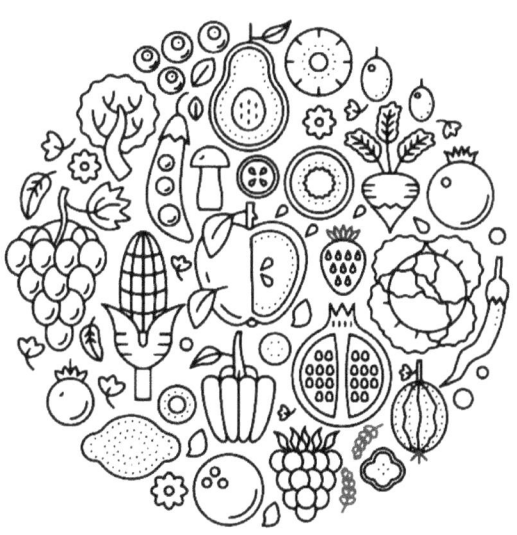

Cooking Essentials for Recipe Success

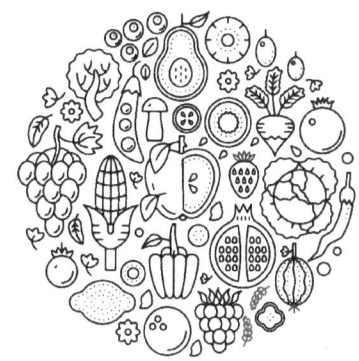

Fruit and Vegetable Preparation
(washing and prepping fruits and vegetables)

Cooking with Beans, Peas, and Lentils
(dried bean preparation, canned bean preparation, bean worksheet)

Cooking Terms
(short list of terms used in the recipes)

Cooking Tools
(list of helpful equipment for cooking)

Name Brands
(brands I often use for ingredients)

Fruit and Vegetable Preparation

Fruits and vegetables should be washed before using for consumption. To do this, place them under cold running water, while rubbing gently or using a clean fruit and vegetable brush. To save on cooking time, many of the fruits and vegetables can be prepped (chopped, diced) in advance and stored in a refrigerator or freezer.

Cooking with Beans, Peas, and Lentils

Dried bean preparation—sorting and soaking:

Before you actually cook dried beans, you must sort and soak them. Start by sorting out any foreign materials such as tiny stones or bad beans that may have found their way into your batch of beans. Next, you will soak them overnight (6-8 hours) at room temperature or heat the beans briefly and allow them to soak while cooling over a shorter period of time. I find that the overnight soaking method results in beans that are more intact with a better appearance and texture. However, in a pinch, the quick soak works just fine. The reasons for soaking beans and discarding the soaking water are to shorten cooking time and improve the digestibility of the beans. Soaking helps to break down the oligosaccharide, lectin, and phytate content naturally present in beans. Oligosaccharides are associated with flatulence, and lectins and phytates can interfere with zinc and iron absorption. Once the beans are soaked by using either soaking method, they are then cooked in the same way.

Choose a soaking method:

1. Overnight (6-8) hour soak, or
2. Quick soak

Overnight soaking method and cooking for dried beans:

Put the dried beans in a stockpot and completely cover the beans with water. Put the lid on the pot and allow the beans to sit at room temperature for 6-8 hours or overnight. Drain and rinse the beans. When ready to cook, cover the beans with a generous amount of fresh water. With the lid in place, bring the pot to a boil and then turn the heat down to a simmer for about 1-2 hours until the beans reach your desired tenderness. Remove the beans from heat, and drain the water from the pot.

Quick soaking method and cooking for dried beans:

Add dried beans to a stockpot, and completely cover the beans with water. Put the lid on the pot and bring it to a boil for 2 minutes. Remove the pot from the heat source and allow it to sit with the lid on for 1 hour. Drain and rinse the beans. When ready to cook the beans, cover the beans with a generous amount of fresh water. With the lid in place, bring the pot to a boil and then turn the heat down to a simmer for about 1-2 hours until the beans reach your desired tenderness. Remove the beans from heat, and drain the water from the pot.

Canned bean preparation:

Canned beans do not require soaking or preliminary cooking if they will be cooked later as part of the recipe preparation. If the recipe does not call for the canned beans to be heated later, then the beans should be boiled for 5-10 minutes to prevent the very low risk of botulism.

Notes:

1. Dried lentils and dried split peas do not require soaking prior to cooking.
2. Beans are best when cooked to a "soft to the bite" consistency that allows them to maintain their shape. Beans will be too hard or too soft if they are under or overcooked.

Bean worksheet—approximate measurement conversions

Dried beans in volume (cups): ½ cup to ½ cup plus 2 teaspoons	Cooked yields: 1½ cups cooked beans
Canned beans weight: 15 ounces (425 grams)	Yields: 1½ cups cooked beans, ½ cup liquid, with sodium added (often the equivalent of about ⅛ teaspoon table salt)
Dried beans weight: 16 ounces (1 pound) 453 grams	Equivalent dried beans in cups: 2 cups

Cooking Terms

My definitions of a few terms:

Dice: cut into cubes, sides measure ¼-inch
Chop: cut into pieces, less precise than dicing
Julienne: cut into thin strips or ⅛ x ⅛ x 1 to 2 inches
Mince: cut or chop into very small pieces

Cooking Tools

Below is a list of cooking tools that are handy for the recipes in this guide.

Baking dishes and pans
Broiler pan set
Glass or ceramic pie pan, 9-inch
Rectangular glass baking dish, 9 x 13-inch
Sheet pan
Solid round pizza pans, 14-inch (2)

Bowls, baskets, and sieves
Colander—mesh
Colander—regular
Stainless steel or glass mixing bowl set
Steamer basket

Cookware set and other pieces (stainless steel or non-stick surfaces will work)
Saucepan (1.5-quart) or fry pan (8-inch)
Saucepans with lids, (2 to 4-quart) (2)
Saute pan with lid, 10-inch or larger depending on the space on your cooktop
Skillet with lid, 10-inch or larger depending on the space on your cooktop
Stockpots with lids, 6-quart or larger (2)

Cutting tools
Cutting board
Fruit and vegetable peeler
Kitchen shears
Knives
       Chef knife
       Paring knife
       Serrated utility or bread knife

Blenders/mixer
Blenders—handheld immersion and countertop stand-alone
Mixer—handheld or stand-alone

Pastry tools
Pastry cutter
Mini pastry or pizza smooth dough roller, or 6-inch mini/small French rolling pin
Silicone pastry brush

Storage containers and labels
Food grade plastic storage containers (different sizes)
Glass storage containers with lids (different sizes)
Masking tape
Sharpie

Utensils
Metal spatula—narrow and regular size
Potato masher
Silicone (side or spoon) spatula—mini and regular size
Stirring spoon—large size
Tongs
Vegetable washing brush
Whisk

Other
Digital kitchen scale

Name Brands

Here are several of the name brands of ingredients that I have used in these recipes. Brand selection can make a difference in how the recipes turn out, but in most cases a suitable substitute brand will also work well.

Beans and peas:
Camellia Brand® Lady Cream Peas (dried)

Bouillon base and cubes:
Better than Bouillon® No Chicken and No Beef Base
Edward & Sons® Not-Chick'n and Not-Beef Bouillon Cubes

Cheese alternative:
Follow Your Heart® Parmesan style—shredded

Butter alternative:
Earth Balance® Vegan Buttery Sticks
Smart Balance® Original Buttery Spread

Sour cream alternative:
Tofutti Brand® Better Than Sour Cream

The Recipes

Supper or Main Meal, Sides, Lunch, Breakfast, Beverages, Desserts

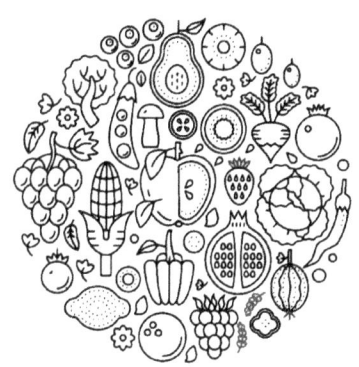

Supper or Main Meal

1. Artichokes with Hollandaise Sauce 77
2. Broccoli and Potato Soup 79
3. Chili de Verduras 81
4. Creamy Corn Chowder 83
5. Down by the Bay Gumbo 85
6. Enchiladas Poblano 87
7. Falafels with Tzatziki Sauce 90
8. Favorite Red Beans and Rice 93
9. French Market Soup 95
10. Garden Wrap 97
11. Lasagna Vegetali 99
12. Lemongrass Ginger Vegetables and Tofu Noodle Bowl 102
13. Lentillies 105
14. Magnificent Macaroni Casserole 107
15. Night on the Mediterranean Gyro 109
16. Old Fashioned Squash Casserole 111
17. Red and White Pizzas 113
18. Savory Spaghetti 116
19. Sesame Garlic Vegetables and Tofu with Rice 118

20 Simple Leek Soup	121
21 Southern Black-eyed Peas	123
22 Spiced Beanloaf	124
23 Spinach and Sweet Pepper Quiche	126
24 Split Pea and Carrot Soup	129
25 Tasty Tacos	130
26 Topside Pot Pie	132
27 Turnip Greens and Dumplings	135
28 Vegetable Divan	137

Sides

1. Buttered Sweet Peas 140
2. Classic Hummus 141
3. Meltaway Cornbread 143
4. Parsley Mashed Potatoes 144
5. Sauteed Asparagus Spears 146
6. Seasonal Fresh Fruit Medley 147
7. Spring Side Salad 148
8. Super Slaw 150
9. Tabouli Salad 151

Lunch

1. Broccoli, Apple, Walnut Salad 153
2. Butter Bean and Corn Salad 154
3. Chickpea Chia Salad 155
4. Crisp Vegetables and Hummus Sandwich 157
5. Lady Pea Salad 159
6. Quinoa Black Bean Bowl with Mango and Kale 160
7. Wild West Dip with Chips 162

Breakfast

1. Bagels with Seed Butter and Berries 165
2. Banana Muffins 166
3. Blueberry Muffins 168

4. Good-Morning Grits 170
5. Heavenly Hash Browns and Black Beans 172
6. Overnight Oats with Peaches 174
7. Perfect Pancakes or Waffles 175

Beverages

1. Strawberry Dream Smoothie 178
2. Sunshine Smoothie 179

Desserts

1. Apple Crisp 181
2. Chocolate Chip Oatmeal Cookies 183

Supper or Main Meal Recipes

Artichokes with Hollandaise Sauce   77
Broccoli and Potato Soup   79
Chili de Verduras   81
Creamy Corn Chowder   83
Down by the Bay Gumbo   85
Enchiladas Poblano   87
Falafels with Tzatziki Sauce   90
Favorite Red Beans and Rice   93
French Market Soup   95
Garden Wrap   97
Lasagna Vegetali   99
Lemongrass Ginger Vegetables and Tofu Noodle Bowl   102
Lentillies   105
Magnificent Macaroni Casserole   107
Night on the Mediterranean Gyro   109
Old Fashioned Squash Casserole   111
Red and White Pizzas   113
Savory Spaghetti   116
Sesame Garlic Vegetables and Tofu with Rice   118
Simple Leek Soup   121
Southern Black-eyed Peas   123
Spiced Beanloaf   124
Spinach and Sweet Pepper Quiche   126
Split Pea and Carrot Soup   129
Tasty Tacos   130
Topside Pot Pie   132
Turnip Greens and Dumplings   135
Vegetable Divan   137

Artichoke with Hollandaise Sauce

"Give me the Biggest Artichoke, Momma!" Artichokes with plant-based Hollandaise Sauce are a favorite at our house. My children started eating artichokes around the age of three. It took a little training for them to be able to get the meat off the artichoke leaf; however, it was a delight to watch that process.

Artichokes

4 artichokes	(1,590 grams)
1 teaspoon (5 milliliters) extra virgin olive oil	(5 grams)
¼ teaspoon table salt	(2 grams)

Hollandaise sauce

½ cup plant butter	(110 grams)
15 ounces canned northern beans with juice, divided	(425 grams)
3 tablespoons plant mayonnaise	(40 grams)
1½ tablespoons (25 milliliters) lemon juice	(25 grams)

For the artichokes: Trim the pointed tips of each artichoke leaf with kitchen shears. Grasp the thick part of the artichoke with one hand, and use a large, sharp, serrated knife in the other hand to cut off and discard the top ¼ portion (opposite the stalk) of the artichoke. Slice off the end of the stalk at an angle.

Add olive oil and salt to a large stockpot (6-quart or larger). Two stockpots may be needed for large artichokes. Place the artichokes in the pot and add water to cover or almost cover the artichokes. Place the lid on the pot. Bring water to a boil and then turn down to a simmer. Cook for 50-60 additional minutes. Remove the artichokes from heat, and drain the water.

For the sauce: While the artichokes are cooking, make the hollandaise sauce. Pour a can of northern beans including the juice into a blender and puree until silky smooth (about 1 minute). Measure out ½ cup of the puree. Freeze the remaining bean puree in ½ cup portions (label and date) for future recipes. In a small saucepan, melt the butter on medium-low. Add ½ cup pureed beans. Cook over low to medium heat for 10 minutes, stirring frequently to prevent sticking. Whisk in the mayonnaise and lemon juice while cooking. Pour the sauce into 4 small custard cups for dipping.

To eat an artichoke, peel off a leaf, dip the meaty part at the base of the leaf in the sauce, and scrape the meaty part off with your teeth. Once you have reached the core, use a butter knife to carefully remove the thistle while leaving the heart or meaty center to eat.

Servings: 4 **Serving size:** 1 artichoke (480 grams), ¼ cup sauce (75 grams)

Recommend with: whole-grain roll, fresh fruit, and plant milk.

Notes:
1. To save time, prepare artichokes and hollandaise sauce ahead of cooking time. After trimming, roll the artichokes in a bowl of lemon juice ensuring that all cut parts are covered by juice to prevent discoloration. Store the artichokes and sauce in the refrigerator. Warm the sauce in a microwave oven just before serving.
2. Shop for artichokes with leaves that are mostly closed which usually indicates greater freshness.
3. There are online videos that demonstrate how to scrape out the thistle and eat the heart of the artichoke.

Nutrients Per Serving: 329 calories, 24 grams fat, 6 grams saturated fat, 8 grams protein, 26 grams carbohydrate, 10 grams fiber, 372 milligrams sodium. Iodized salt and olive oil used in water for artichokes were not included in estimations.

Broccoli and Potato Soup

This recipe is quick to make, tasty, and filling. It makes quite a bit, so expect leftovers. One trick for reducing strong aromas, such as those given off by cooking cruciferous vegetables, is to light a candle.

½ cup plus 2 teaspoons dried navy beans or 15 ounces canned, drained	(110 grams)
3½ cups (830 milliliters) water, divided	(830 grams)
1 tablespoon plant chicken flavor bouillon base or cubes for 3 cup equivalent, do not reconstitute	(20 grams)
½ cup nutritional yeast	(40 grams)
½ teaspoon table salt	(3 grams)
½ teaspoon black pepper	(1 gram)
8 cups fresh broccoli florets with 2-inch stems	(730 grams)
2 cups chopped (½-inch sides) yellow or sweet onions	(320 grams)
2 cups potato chunks (¾-inch sides) with skin from about 2 potatoes, 2 by 4 inches each	(350 grams)
¼ cup plant butter	(55 grams)
1 cup (240 milliliters) unsweetened soymilk	(240 grams)

For dried beans, use the overnight or quick soaking method to prepare the beans. Drain and then immerse beans in plenty of fresh water in a large covered pot. Bring to a boil and turn down to a simmer for 1½ hours until the beans are tender. Remove from heat, drain, and cool. Refrigerate beans that will not be used at this time.

Canned beans should be drained but not soaked or cooked.

Using a blender, puree the navy beans with ½ cup water to a silky-smooth consistency and set aside.

Add 3 cups of water, bouillon base, nutritional yeast, salt, and pepper to a large stockpot. Cover and bring to a simmer. Add broccoli and onions. Cover and simmer for 10 minutes. Remove the pot from heat, and use a hand blender to create a rough puree containing small pieces of broccoli.

Supper or Main Meal Recipes | 79

Add the bean puree and potato chunks to the stockpot containing the broccoli. Heat to a strong simmer, and cook for 10-15 minutes, stirring occasionally. Add plant butter and soymilk and simmer for 1 additional minute before serving.

Servings: 10 **Serving size:** 1 cup (250 grams)

Recommend with: whole-grain bread, fresh fruit, and plant milk.

Notes:
1. Cut onions and broccoli ahead of cooking time.
2. Leftovers may be refrigerated.

Nutrients Per Serving: 149 calories, 4 grams fat, 1 gram saturated fat, 7 grams protein, 21 grams carbohydrate, 6 grams fiber, 377 milligrams sodium

Chili de Verduras

Use this wonderful recipe to feed a crowd or keep in your freezer to pull out for quick meals. Dark red kidney beans or light red kidney beans will both work here. Add extra chili powder, hot sauce, or salt to individual servings as desired. Plan to receive compliments from hungry customers!

1 cup plus 4 teaspoons dried red kidney beans or 30 ounces canned, drained	(200 grams)
2 cups peeled and chopped (½-inch sides) celery lightly peel tough outer layer	(200 grams)
2 cups chopped (½-inch sides) yellow or sweet onions	(320 grams)
1 cup dried common brown lentils, rinsed	(190 grams)
5 cups (1,180 milliliters) water	(1,180 grams)
29 ounces canned diced tomatoes	(820 grams)
12 ounces canned tomato paste	(340 grams)
⅓ cup chili powder	(40 grams)
1 tablespoon minced garlic	(9 grams)
2 teaspoons plant beef flavor bouillon base or cubes for 2 cup equivalent, do not reconstitute	(10 grams)
1 teaspoon table salt	(6 grams)
2 cups frozen cut corn	(330 grams)

Toppings (make fresh in the amount needed for each meal)
servings below are for a 4-person meal

¼ cup sliced (¼-inch thick rounds) scallions	(25 grams)
¼ cup shredded plant cheddar cheese	(30 grams)
¼ cup plant sour cream	(55 grams)

Soak dried kidney beans overnight or for 6-8 hours in a stockpot with a generous covering of water. Drain soaking water. Cover with plenty of fresh water and bring to a boil. Turn down to a strong simmer for 1 hour. Remove from heat and drain. See notes if using canned beans.

In a 6-quart or larger stockpot, add the cooked dry beans, celery, onions, lentils, and the remaining chili ingredients except for the frozen corn and canned beans (see notes if using) to the pot. Bring to a boil and then turn down to a simmer, stirring occasionally to prevent sticking to the bottom of the pot. Simmer for 45 minutes. Add corn and, (if using) drained canned beans (see notes) during the final 15 minutes of cooking.

Servings: 13 **Serving size:** 1 cup (250 grams) chili, 1 tablespoon each topping (30 grams)

Recommend with: saltines or tortilla chips, Spring Side Salad, fresh fruit, and plant milk.

Notes:
1. To save on cooking time, peel and chop celery and onions in advance. Store in the refrigerator or freezer.
2. Try using a pre-minced garlic to save time.
3. If using canned beans, drain and add with the corn during the last 15 minutes of cooking time.
4. For leftovers, allow chili to cool down. Divide it into portions sized according to your meal needs and pour into glass or plastic food-grade containers. Label, date, and freeze.
5. Consider browning a small amount of ground turkey meat to add to individual servings for non-plant-based eaters. You may also use regular cheese or Greek yogurt for toppings.

Nutrients Per Serving: 245 calories, 5 grams fat, 2 grams saturated fat, 12 grams protein, 43 grams carbohydrate, 12 grams fiber, 682 milligrams sodium

Creamy Corn Chowder

This easy and delicious recipe makes quite a bit, and it freezes well for leftovers. My favorite variety of corn for this recipe is White Shoepeg.

1 cup dried red lentils, rinsed	(190 grams)
2½ cups frozen cut white or yellow corn kernels, divided	(310 grams)
1 cup chopped (½-inch sides) yellow or sweet onions	(170 grams)
¼ cup nutritional yeast	(20 grams)
4 teaspoons plant chicken flavor bouillon base or cubes for 4 cup equivalent, do not reconstitute	(25 grams)
¼ teaspoon table salt	(2 grams)
¼ teaspoon black pepper	(1 gram)
3½ cups (830 milliliters) water, divided	(830 grams)
½ cup sliced (¼-inch thick rounds) carrots	(65 grams)
2 cups (470 milliliters) unsweetened coconut milk refrigerated or boxed type, not canned, about 60 calories per cup	(460 grams)
¼ cup plant butter	(55 grams)

Add lentils, 2 cups corn, onions, nutritional yeast, bouillon, salt, pepper, and 3 cups water to a stockpot (6-quart or larger). With the lid on, bring to a boil and turn down to a simmer for 20 additional minutes. Remove from heat. Using a hand blender, puree ingredients in the stockpot until smooth.

In a separate small saucepan, add the remaining ½ cup corn, carrots, and ½ cup water. With the lid on, bring to a boil and turn down to a simmer for another 20 minutes.

Add the corn and carrots mix, milk, and butter to the large stockpot. Cover and heat to a simmer for 5 minutes. Stir and scrape the bottom of the pot every minute to prevent chowder from sticking there.

Servings: 9   **Serving size:** 1 cup (250 grams)

Recommend with: whole-grain bread, fresh fruit, and plant milk.

Notes:
1. Consider chopping the onions and carrots ahead of time.

Nutrients Per Serving: 188 calories, 6 grams fat, 2 grams saturated fat, 8 grams protein, 26 grams carbohydrate, 4 grams fiber, 422 milligrams sodium

Down by the Bay Gumbo

One of the secrets of great gumbo is to start with a dark brown roux. Although it takes a little time to make, this gumbo is worth it, and the recipe makes enough for more than one meal. Hot pepper sauce lovers will enjoy adding a few drops to their bowl.

½ cup plus 2 teaspoons dried pinto beans	(100 grams)
¼ cup (60 milliliters) canola oil	(55 grams)
¼ cup all-purpose flour	(30 grams)
½ cup peeled and chopped (½-inch sides) celery lightly peel tough outer layer	(50 grams)
½ cup chopped (½-inch sides) green bell peppers	(75 grams)
½ cup chopped (½-inch sides) yellow or sweet onions	(80 grams)
6 cups (1,420 milliliters) water	(1,420 grams)
2 tablespoons (30 milliliters) white vinegar	(30 grams)
2 tablespoons (30 milliliters) less sodium soy sauce	(30 grams)
1 tablespoon plant chicken flavor bouillon base or cubes for 3 cup equivalent, do not reconstitute	(20 grams)
14.5 ounces canned diced tomatoes	(410 grams)
¼ cup finely chopped fresh parsley	(15 grams)
2 teaspoons minced garlic	(6 grams)
½ teaspoon table salt	(3 grams)
¼ teaspoon ground red pepper	(<1 gram)
½ cup dry brown rice	(90 grams)
½ cup dried common brown lentils, rinsed	(100 grams)
1 tablespoon gumbo file	(4 grams)
12 ounces (3¼ cups) frozen cut okra	(340 grams)

Prepare the pinto beans by using the overnight soak method. Discard soaking water. Add fresh water and bring pinto beans to a boil. Turn the heat down to a simmer for 1 hour. Drain the beans and set aside.

For the roux, add canola oil to a saucepan. Turn heat to medium or medium-high. Add flour. Stir continuously and adjust heat to prevent sticking and burning while bringing to a strong simmer. Turn heat down to medium or medium-low keeping a strong simmer while stirring continuously for about 20-25 minutes until the roux has turned a rich dark brown color (not caramel or medium brown color). Do not burn or you will need to start over. Remove from heat and continue to stir for a few minutes. Set aside.

Add pinto beans, roux, celery, bell peppers, onions, water, vinegar, soy sauce, bouillon, tomatoes, parsley, garlic, salt, pepper, rice, and lentils to a large stockpot (6-quart or larger). Sprinkle around the gumbo file. Stir all until combined.

Bring to a boil (covered) and quickly turn heat down to a simmer. After 15 minutes of simmering, add okra. Continue simmer (covered) for 30 minutes.

Servings: 11 **Serving size:** 1 cup (240 grams)

Recommend with: whole-grain French roll, fresh fruit, and plant milk.

Notes:
1. Cut celery, bell peppers, onions, and parsley ahead of time and store in the refrigerator.
2. Make roux ahead of time and store in the refrigerator to make cooking time go faster. Switch hands while stirring roux to prevent fatigue.
3. Freeze leftover portions for a future meal. Measure out the amount needed per meal and place into separate containers. Label, date, and freeze once cooled.
4. To please non-plant-based eaters, bake about 8 ounces of whitefish. Shred and add to individual servings or to half the pot of gumbo in the last 15 minutes of cooking.

Nutrients Per Serving: 171 calories, 5 grams fat, 0 grams saturated fat, 6 grams protein, 25 grams carbohydrate, 6 grams fiber, 432 milligrams sodium

Enchiladas Poblano

This plant-based version of classic enchiladas is great to feed groups. It can be prepared ahead of time, frozen without the white sauce and salsa toppings and thawed overnight in the refrigerator before baking. Double the recipe as needed to feed more people.

Bean filling

1 cup plus 4 teaspoons dried pinto beans	(210 grams)
or 30 ounces canned, drained	
½ cup (120 milliliters) water	(120 grams)
1 teaspoon plant chicken flavor bouillon base	(6 grams)
or cube for 1 cup equivalent, do not reconstitute	

Vegetable filling

1 cup julienne sliced poblano peppers	(85 grams)
from about 1 large or 2 medium size peppers	
1 cup julienne sliced yellow or sweet onions	(160 grams)
¼ teaspoon table salt	(2 grams)
Cooking spray	

White sauce

1 cup (240 milliliters) unsweetened coconut milk, divided	(230 grams)
refrigerated or boxed type, not canned, about 60 calories per cup	
1 teaspoon plant chicken flavor bouillon base	(6 grams)
or cube for 1 cup equivalent, do not reconstitute	
1 tablespoon cornstarch	(8 grams)
2 teaspoons nutritional yeast	(3 grams)
⅛ teaspoon table salt	(1 gram)

Tortillas and toppings

8 (8-inch) flour tortillas	(370 grams)
1 cup halved grape or cherry tomatoes	(180 grams)
2 medium Hass avocados, sliced in strips lengthwise (see Note 1)	(270 grams)
½ cup prepared mild salsa	(120 grams)

For the beans: For dried beans, use the overnight or quick soaking method to prepare the beans. Drain and then immerse beans in plenty of fresh water in a large covered pot. Bring to a boil and turn down to a simmer for 1½-2 hours until the beans are mashably soft. Remove from heat, drain, and cool. Refrigerate beans that will not be used at this time.

Canned beans should be drained but not soaked or cooked.

For the bean filling: Mix ½ cup water with bouillon base. Place in a microwave safe bowl, cover, and heat for 15-20 seconds to dissolve bouillon. Pour over beans. Use a potato masher or hand blender on the bean mix to produce a lumpy smooth consistency. Set aside.

For the vegetable filling: Spray a large skillet with cooking spray. Place sliced peppers and onions in the skillet, turn heat to medium, and cook until tender (about 15-20 minutes). Sprinkle with salt. Set aside.

For the white sauce: Whisk together ½ cup coconut milk, bouillon base, and cornstarch powder in a bowl until dissolved. Add the remaining milk, nutritional yeast, and salt. Pour into a saucepan. Use a spatula to remove any remaining ingredients from the bowl. Heat (covered) just to a boil and then turn down to medium-low, stirring constantly until thickened (about 2 minutes). Remove from heat and set aside.

For the tortillas and toppings: Spray a 9 x 13-inch glass baking dish with cooking spray. Add about ¼ cup bean filling and about 2 tablespoons vegetable filling to the center of 8 tortillas. Leave 1 inch on the end of each tortilla free of filling. Roll tortillas into cylinders and line them up side by side in the baking dish.

Bake tortillas in 350°F (177°C) oven for 20 minutes, uncovered. Wash and half tomatoes, and set aside. Measure out salsa and set aside. After 20 minutes, add tomatoes evenly on top of tortillas. Cook for another 10 minutes.

Using a paring knife, slice 1 or 2 avocados (see Note 1) lengthwise into quarters, hitting the seed with each slice. Use the knife as a wedge between slices to release the pieces. Remove the seed and outer skin. If not using all 8 servings of enchiladas for this meal, slice only 1 avocado because avocados lose freshness once opened.

Cover the white sauce and reheat in a microwave oven for about 20-30 seconds. Drizzle the white sauce over the enchiladas at serving time to avoid sogginess.

Spoon 1 tablespoon of salsa over each enchilada, and place avocado slices on the side of each serving.

Servings: 8   **Serving size:** 1 enchilada (240 grams)

Recommend with: corn, brown rice, or black beans, fresh fruit, and plant milk.

Notes:
1. Slice avocados close to serving time to avoid discoloration. Sprinkle avocado slices with lemon or lime juice if not eating immediately to prevent discoloration. Watch a how-to video from the internet to observe how to slice an avocado as needed.
2. To satisfy non-plant-based eaters, sprinkle half enchiladas with shredded cheese and chicken.

Nutrients Per Serving: 321 calories, 10 grams fat, 2 grams saturated fat, 11 grams protein, 49 grams carbohydrate, 10 grams fiber, 717 milligrams sodium

Falafels with Tzatziki Sauce

These falafels are crisp on the outside and savory on the inside. Great side items with falafels are a simple salad with cucumber slices, lettuce, and tomato (no recipe needed), or my Sauteed Asparagus recipe. Falafels freeze well for a future meal.

Falafels

1 cup dried chickpeas, use only dried chickpeas	(200 grams)
1 cup (240 milliliters) unsweetened coconut milk, divided	(230 grams)
refrigerated or boxed type, not canned, about 60 calories per cup	
¼ cup all-purpose flour	(30 grams)
1 tablespoon black chia seeds	(10 grams)
1 cup diced (¼-inch sides) yellow or sweet onions	(160 grams)
Cooking spray	
¼ cup large-grated lemon rind	(25 grams)
1 teaspoon minced garlic	(3 grams)
1 teaspoon table salt	(6 grams)
⅛ teaspoon cumin	(<1 gram)
⅛ teaspoon ground red pepper	(<1 gram)
1¼ cups panko bread crumbs	(65 grams)
½ cup (120 milliliters) canola oil, divided	(110 grams)
Lemon wedges, deseeded (optional)	
Parsley twigs for garnish (optional)	

Tzatziki sauce

¾ cup peeled, diced (¼-inch sides) English cucumber	(100 grams)
¼ teaspoon table salt, divided	(2 grams)
¾ cup plant sour cream	(170 grams)
⅛ teaspoon dried dill weed	(<1 gram)
1 teaspoon minced garlic	(3 grams)
2 tablespoons (30 milliliters) lemon juice	(30 grams)

For the falafels: Prepare chickpeas by using the overnight or quick soak method. Drain and then cover with plenty of fresh water. Bring to a boil and then turn down to a simmer for 1½-2 hours. Drain and set aside.

Make a thick white sauce by whisking together ½ cup of coconut milk and flour. Work out any lumps, then whisk in the remaining coconut milk. Heat sauce in a small saucepan on medium heat, stirring occasionally to prevent sauce from sticking to the bottom. Once sauce has thickened, remove from heat. Stir in black chia seeds and allow to cool.

Puree together the cooked chickpeas and the thick white sauce until the puree is lumpy smooth. An immersion blender works well for this. Set aside.

Spray a saute pan with cooking spray. Cook onions on medium to medium-low heat for about 20 minutes until the juices cook out. Turn heat down if onions begin to burn. Set aside.

Chop large grated lemon rinds a bit more. Combine chickpeas, onions, lemon rind, garlic, salt, cumin, and pepper together. Refrigerate until ready to cook.

Place panko crumbs in a bowl. Scoop out ¼ cup chickpea mixture and form into a ball. Roll in the panko crumbs until fully covered. Continue to scoop and roll until all chickpea mixture is used.

Select the falafels needed for this meal. Refrigerate or freeze the remainder for a future meal (see Note 5).

Prepare and chill the tzatziki sauce (see below).

Spread 2 tablespoons of canola oil in a large saute pan or skillet, and heat to medium-high. When the oil is heated, place 4-5 falafels at a time in the pan. Turn down heat to medium. Cook uncovered for 5 minutes or until golden brown. Turn down the heat a little more if falafels are burning. Carefully turn falafels once using a large spoon, and cook for another 5 minutes or until golden brown. Keep cooked falafels warm in a 250°F (121°C) oven.

When ready to cook another batch, add 2 more tablespoons of canola oil to the pan. Allow the oil to heat before adding the falafels.

For the tzatziki sauce: Place peeled and diced cucumber in a strainer. Sprinkle with ⅛ teaspoon of salt, and toss to distribute evenly. Allow the cucumber to sit in the strainer for 20 minutes. Rinse. Squeeze excess water from the cucumber with the back of a spoon and paper towels, and place cucumber in a bowl. If using the pre-minced variety, squeeze garlic with the back of a spoon to remove excess liquid. Add sour cream, dill weed, ⅛ teaspoon salt, garlic, and lemon juice to the cucumber, and stir together. Place in the refrigerator to chill.

To serve, add 1 tablespoon of chilled sauce to a hot falafel. Garnish with lemon wedges and sprigs of fresh parsley.

Servings: 8 (makes 16 falafels)   **Serving size:** 2 falafels (120 grams) and 2 tablespoons of sauce (30 grams)

Recommend with: English cucumber slices with lettuce and tomato, quinoa, fresh fruit, and plant milk.

Notes:
1. Almond milk or another plant milk may be used in place of coconut milk.
2. Try using pre-minced garlic to save time.
3. Cook chickpeas in advance and refrigerate.
4. To save time, make tzatziki sauce a day ahead of cooking time and refrigerate.
5. To use frozen falafels, allow them to thaw overnight in the refrigerator and begin at the next step (cooking in canola oil).

Nutrients Per Serving: 332 calories, 20 grams fat, 3 grams saturated fat, 7 grams protein, 33 grams carbohydrate, 6 grams fiber, 450 milligrams sodium

Favorite Red Beans and Rice

This warm and filling recipe makes many servings. It will be a hit at your next tailgate or other gathering and will have people coming back for more. Top individual servings with a little plant-based sour cream as desired.

1½ cups plus 2 tablespoons dried red kidney beans	(300 grams)
6¼ cups (1,480 milliliters) water, divided	(1,480 grams)
2 cups chopped (½-inch sides) yellow or sweet onions	(320 grams)
1 cup peeled and chopped (½-inch sides) celery lightly peel tough outer layer	(100 grams)
1 cup chopped (½-inch sides) green bell peppers	(150 grams)
1 cup chopped (½-inch sides) red bell peppers	(150 grams)
½ cup chopped fresh cilantro, divided	(8 grams)
2 teaspoons minced garlic	(6 grams)
2 teaspoons (10 milliliters) less sodium soy sauce	(10 grams)
2 teaspoons plant chicken flavor bouillon base or cubes for 2 cup equivalent, do not reconstitute	(10 grams)
2 teaspoons plant beef flavor bouillon base or cubes for 2 cup equivalent, do not reconstitute	(10 grams)
⅛ teaspoon paprika	(<1 gram)
⅛ teaspoon ground red pepper	(<1 gram)
⅛ teaspoon table salt	(1 gram)
1½ cups dry brown rice	(280 grams)
1 tablespoon all-purpose flour	(8 grams)
2 tablespoons (30 milliliters) extra virgin olive oil	(25 grams)

Soak dried kidney beans overnight or for 6-8 hours in a stockpot with a generous covering of water. Drain soaking water. Refrigerate beans until cooking time.

Wash and chop onions, celery, bell peppers, and cilantro. Set aside.

Place beans in a large stockpot and add 6 cups of water. Cover with lid and bring to a simmer for 10 minutes. During initial simmer, add garlic, soy sauce, bouillon, paprika, red pepper, and salt to the stockpot. In a small bowl, whisk together flour and ¼ cup cool water until smooth. After beans have simmered for 10 minutes add flour mix, onions, celery, bell peppers, ¼ cup cilantro, and rice to the stockpot. Replace the stockpot lid and continue to simmer for 50 more minutes

(60 minutes total). Stir occasionally to prevent sticking to the bottom of the pot. Mix in the olive oil at the end of cooking.

Sprinkle remaining fresh cilantro on each serving.

Servings: 11   **Serving size:** 1 cup (250 grams)

Recommend with: whole-grain French roll or bread, fresh fruit, and plant milk.

Notes:
1. Prepare vegetables ahead of cooking time and store in the refrigerator.
2. Assemble seasonings, wet and dry together, ahead of time in a small glass bowl. Cover and store in the refrigerator until cooking time. Ensure all ingredients are removed from the bowl by using a spatula and a tablespoon or two of water.
3. Add a small amount of sausage to individual servings for meat lovers.

Nutrients Per Serving: 234 calories, 4 grams fat, 1 gram saturated fat, 9 grams protein, 42 grams carbohydrate, 9 grams fiber, 327 milligrams sodium

French Market Soup

This handy recipe takes little time in the kitchen, and it makes a lot. If a red chili pepper is not available, an easy substitute is ⅛ teaspoon ground red pepper.

2 cups dried variety beans	(380 grams)
8 cups (1,890 milliliters) of water	(1,890 grams)
29 ounces canned diced tomatoes	(820 grams)
1 cup chopped (¾-inch sides) yellow or sweet onions	(160 grams)
¼ cup (60 milliliters) lemon juice	(60 grams)
2 tablespoons diced (¼-inch sides) red chili peppers	(20 grams)
1 tablespoon plant chicken flavor bouillon base or cubes for 3 cup equivalent, do not reconstitute	(20 grams)
2 teaspoons (10 milliliters) less sodium soy sauce	(10 grams)
1 teaspoon minced garlic	(3 grams)
½ teaspoon table salt	(3 grams)
¼ teaspoon black pepper	(1 gram)

Soak beans overnight or for 6-8 hours in a stockpot with a generous covering of water. Drain soaking water. Refrigerate beans that you are not using right away.

When ready to cook, add 8 cups fresh water to the beans in a large stockpot and bring to a boil. Turn down to a simmer. Add all of the remaining ingredients. Simmer (covered) for 2-3 hours or until beans are tender.

Servings: 14   **Serving size:** 1 cup (240 grams)

Recommend with: whole-grain baguette or roll, fresh fruit, and plant milk.

Notes:
1. Chop onions and dice chili peppers ahead of time.
2. Wear gloves when working with the chili peppers if your skin is sensitive.
3. Try pre-minced garlic to save time.
4. Double recipe ingredients, and freeze leftovers in 4-serving containers for quick meals.
5. For non-plant-based eaters, consider placing a little ground turkey meat or sausage on the side for individuals to add.

Nutrients Per Serving: 123 calories, 1 gram fat, 0 grams saturated fat, 7 grams protein, 23 grams carbohydrate, 7 grams fiber, 366 milligrams sodium

Garden Wrap

This fresh and tasty wrap recipe goes well with your favorite plant-based Italian or ranch dressing. Soft spinach or tomato tortillas are healthy choices that taste great in this recipe. Add fresh fruit and an avocado slice on the side to make a beautiful plate, and "Wow", what a wrap!

½ cup plus 2 teaspoons dried northern beans or 15 ounces canned	(100 grams)
3 cups torn (1-inch pieces) green leaf lettuce	(70 grams)
1 cup peeled and chopped (½-inch sides) cucumber from about ½ large English cucumber	(130 grams)
1 cup chopped (½-inch sides) tomato	(180 grams)
2 tablespoons diced (¼-inch sides) purple onions	(20 grams)
½ cup (120 milliliters) plant-based Italian or ranch dressing	(120 grams)
¼ teaspoon table salt	(2 grams)
⅛ teaspoon black pepper	(<1 grams)
1 cup crunched (½-inch pieces) plant croutons	(55 grams)
4 (10-inch) spinach or tomato tortillas	(280 grams)

Soak dried northern beans overnight or for 6-8 hours in a stockpot with a generous covering of water. Drain soaking water. Cover beans with plenty of fresh water and bring to a boil. Turn down to a strong simmer for 1½-2 hours until the beans are tender. Remove from heat, drain, and cool. Refrigerate beans that will not be used at this time.

For canned beans, bring beans with liquid to a boil and turn down to a simmer for 5 minutes. Remove from heat, drain and allow to cool. Refrigerate the cooled beans if using them later.

Combine beans, lettuce, cucumber, tomato, onions, dressing, salt, and pepper in a large mixing bowl. Mix by hand to distribute ingredients uniformly.

Crunch large croutons into ½-inch pieces by placing the croutons in a plastic bag and lightly hitting them with a rolling pin. Add the croutons to the vegetable mixture just before serving.

Place ¼ of vegetable mixture in the center of a large tortilla. Pull one side of the tortilla over the vegetable mixture, and tuck it under the tortilla on the other side so that you can tightly roll the mixture up into a snug and secure cylindrical shape that is open at both ends. Diagonally, cut the tortilla in half. Repeat the process with the remaining 3 tortillas.

Servings: 4	**Serving size:** 1 wrap (280 grams)

Recommend with: avocado slices, fresh fruit, and plant milk.

Notes:
1. Tear lettuce and chop onions ahead of time. Store separately in the refrigerator.
2. Crunch the croutons and store in a dry sealed container until ready to use.
3. Easily please non-plant-based eaters with a little chicken breast meat added to individual servings.

Nutrients Per Serving: 438 calories, 14 grams fat, 3 grams saturated fat, 14 grams protein, 64 grams carbohydrate, 7 grams fiber, 799 milligrams sodium

Lasagna Vegetali

Need a crowd pleaser to feed a group? This one will do the trick. Have little time to prepare meals on certain days? This recipe freezes well for later use when time is limited.

Field peas and mushroom layer

1½ cups plus 2 teaspoons frozen black-eyed peas	(215 grams)
8 ounces diced (¼-inch sides) baby bella mushrooms	(230 grams)
Cooking spray	
2 teaspoons plant beef flavor bouillon base or cubes for 2 cup equivalent, do not reconstitute	(10 grams)
1 teaspoon dried basil	(1 gram)
¼ teaspoon table salt	(2 grams)

Cauliflower layer

6 cups chopped cauliflower florets	(700 grams)
1 cup chopped (½-inch sides) yellow or sweet onions	(160 grams)
1½ teaspoons dried oregano	(2 grams)
½ teaspoon minced garlic	(1 gram)
½ teaspoon table salt	(3 grams)
¾ cup plant mayonnaise	(170 grams)

Noodles

1 teaspoon (5 milliliters) extra virgin olive oil	(5 grams)
8 whole-grain lasagna noodles	(200 grams)

Sauce and topping

24 ounces jarred spaghetti or marinara sauce	(750 grams)
14.5 ounces canned diced tomatoes, divided	(410 grams)
¼ cup shredded plant parmesan cheese	(30 grams)

For the field peas and mushroom layer: Cook frozen black-eyed peas in simmering water until soft (about 45 minutes) and drain. Dice mushrooms and set aside. Add the bouillon base, basil, and salt to the cooked peas. Mash with a potato masher to a lumpy consistency. Spray a large saute pan with cooking spray. Add diced mushrooms to the pan and cook over medium heat for about 20 minutes to reduce water. Combine mushrooms with peas and set aside.

For the cauliflower layer: Add cauliflower and onions to a saucepan with enough water to cover vegetables and bring to a boil. Turn down to a simmer for 20 minutes or until soft and mashable. Thoroughly drain excess water. Add oregano, garlic, and salt. Blend with an immersion blender or potato masher until lumpy smooth. Stir in mayonnaise and set aside.

For the noodles: In a large stockpot half full of water, add olive oil, and bring to a boil. Add lasagna noodles to the pot and boil for 8 minutes or according to the package directions. Rinse noodles under cold water. Drain and spread noodles on a cotton kitchen towel avoiding overlap. Pat noodles dry.

To assemble: Assembly is done in layers.
1. Spray a 9 x 13-inch baking dish with cooking spray.
2. Spread ½ cup spaghetti sauce on the bottom of the baking dish.
3. Place 4 noodles side by side on top of sauce.
4. In multiple spots add a total of 1 cup spaghetti sauce on top of noodles, and spread lightly with the back of a spoon.
5. Spoon ½ can of diced tomatoes evenly over the spaghetti sauce layer.
6. Add the mushroom peas in a layer of evenly spaced dollops.
7. Layer the remaining noodles.
8. Dot and softly spread 2 cups of cauliflower sauce.
9. Add the remaining spaghetti sauce, evenly covering all noodles.
10. Dot and spread the rest of the cauliflower sauce. Cover all noodles.
11. Evenly spoon out the remaining half of the diced tomatoes. Cover all noodles.
12. Sprinkle parmesan cheese on top.

Bake uncovered at 350°F (177°C) for 1 hour. Remove from the oven and allow to sit for 10 minutes to solidify. Cut gently with a sharp knife into 12 rectangular servings.

Servings: 12   **Serving size:** 1 rectangular piece (200 grams)

Recommend with: whole-grain ciabatta bread, salad, fresh fruit, and plant milk.

Notes:
1. Chop cauliflower and onions ahead of cooking time. Store in the refrigerator.
2. Use parchment paper followed by plastic wrap or aluminum foil for covering lasagna ahead of baking time. Aluminum foil may react with the acid in the tomato sauce. Uncooked lasagna may be frozen for a few days in advance of baking and eating. Thaw overnight in the refrigerator prior to baking.

3. Freeze baked leftover portions for a future meal. Label, date, and freeze once cooled.
4. To please non-plant-based eaters consider topping part of the lasagna with mozzarella cheese and seasoned ground turkey.

Nutrients Per Serving: 213 calories, 6 grams fat, 1 gram saturated fat, 8 grams protein, 33 grams carbohydrate, 7 grams fiber, 705 milligrams sodium

Lemongrass Ginger Vegetables and Tofu Noodle Bowl

This recipe is an Asian style noodle bowl that is fresh and tasty. A plant-based spring roll on the side goes well with this dish. Add a tiny pinch of ground red pepper to individual servings for those who prefer a little heat.

Tofu

14 ounces drained firm tofu block	(400 grams)
1 tablespoon (15 milliliters) canola oil	(15 grams)
1 tablespoon cornstarch	(8 grams)
Cooking spray	

Sauce

2 cups (470 milliliters) water	(470 grams)
1 tablespoon (15 milliliters) lime juice	(15 grams)
2 teaspoons granulated sugar	(8 grams)
2 teaspoons plant chicken flavor bouillon base or cubes for 2 cup equivalent, do not reconstitute	(10 grams)
1 teaspoon minced garlic	(3 grams)
½ teaspoon table salt	(3 grams)
1 tablespoon minced lemongrass stalk, or paste	(5 grams)
2 teaspoons ginger root zest or paste	(4 grams)
2 teaspoons cornstarch	(5 grams)

Noodles

4 cups (950 milliliters) water	(950 grams)
4 ounces dry brown rice noodles	(110 grams)

Vegetables

2 tablespoons sliced (¼-inch thick rounds) scallions	(10 grams)
1 cup julienne or matchstick sliced carrots	(100 grams)
3 cups (5 ounces dry weight) shredded cabbage	(140 grams)
1 cup snow peas cut in half or thirds on bias tips and edges trimmed	(80 grams)
Cooking spray	
2 teaspoons (10 milliliters) canola oil, divided	(9 grams)

For the tofu: Begin preparing tofu 1-4 hours ahead of cooking time. Unwrap tofu and drain the liquid. Place tofu on a cutting surface. Use a long, smooth, sharp knife to cut the tofu horizontally into two equal pieces that look like two slices of bread in a sandwich. Individually wrap both pieces completely with dry paper towels. Next, wrap the tofu (already in paper towels) with a thin, clean and dry dish towel. Place the wrapped tofu on a plate, and place another plate on top of the tofu with sufficient weight to compress the tofu and drain excess moisture. Refrigerate for 30 minutes. Replace the towels with fresh paper and cloth, and compress for another 20 minutes in the refrigerator.

For the sauce: Add water, lime juice, sugar, bouillon, garlic, and salt to a saucepan (or holding container if making ahead of time). Use a pre-made lemongrass paste or mince a lemongrass stalk. To mince lemongrass, first cut off the ends of the lemongrass stalk and discard. Then peel the outer layer from the stalk and discard. Using a chef's knife, mince the lemongrass stalk, and add to the saucepan. Add ginger paste or fresh ginger root to the saucepan. When using fresh ginger root, peel (and discard) the outer layer of a small piece of ginger with a paring knife and then use a zesting tool to finely grate. Slowly whisk together all the sauce ingredients, except the cornstarch. Dip about ¼ cup of sauce into a separate bowl and whisk in the cornstarch. Add the cornstarch mixture to the rest of the sauce and stir. Cover saucepan, bring to a boil and quickly reduce to a simmer. Stir frequently, and remove from heat once it has thickened a little.

For the noodles: Follow package directions for heat and cooking time. Add water to a stockpot and bring to a boil. Add noodles, cover, and boil according to the package directions. Do not overcook. Drain and rinse under cold water until slightly cooled to prevent noodles from sticking together. Toss and spray with cooking spray to further prevent noodles from sticking together. Set aside.

For the vegetables: Prepare and chop all vegetables. Keep vegetables separated. Reserve scallions for topping just before serving. Spray a large saute pan with cooking spray. Add 1 teaspoon canola oil to the pan. Turn heat to medium-high, and saute carrots for 5 minutes. Next, add cabbage and saute with carrots for 3 minutes. Place cabbage and carrots in a bowl and set aside. Add another 1 teaspoon canola oil to the pan, and saute snow peas for 3 minutes. Place peas in the bowl with cabbage and carrots and set aside.

For the tofu: Retrieve tofu from the refrigerator and carefully remove all wrappings. Combine cornstarch and canola oil to make a paste. Spread the paste evenly over all surfaces of the tofu (a silicone pastry brush works well for this task). Save remaining cornstarch and oil paste for later use. Spray cooking spray on a large saute or fry pan and heat to medium or medium-high heat. Once the pan is hot, add both pieces of tofu side-by-side. Heat for 5 minutes or until tofu begins to turn golden. Carefully flip to the other side for 5 minutes or until tofu starts to turn golden. Now turn the tofu pieces together on each of their four sides and cook for a few minutes until golden. Take the tofu out of the pan onto a cutting board. Using a serrated knife, cut both pieces lengthwise. Brush the newly cut surfaces with the cornstarch and oil paste. Place all pieces back into the pan on the newly cut side that hasn't been cooked and cook for a minute or until golden. Place tofu back on the cutting board, and cut the tofu into 1-inch pieces. Brush the cornstarch and oil paste on the newly cut area and heat those surfaces. Remove the pan from heat, but keep the tofu in the pan until ready to serve. Don't let it sit too long to avoid having it become chewy.

When ready to serve, divide the noodles into individual serving bowls. Spray a saute pan with cooking spray and turn heat to medium-high. When hot, add the mixture of cabbage, carrots, and snow peas to the pan for 1-2 minutes, stirring frequently. Add vegetables over the noodles, and then add tofu to each serving bowl. Shortly before serving, reheat the sauce to a low boil, stir, and pour into each serving bowl. Top each noodle bowl with a sprinkle of green scallions.

Servings: 4   **Serving size:** 1 bowl or ¼ of all ingredients (740 grams)

Recommend with: spring roll, fresh fruit, and plant milk.

Notes:
1. To make the cooking time go more quickly, chop all vegetables ahead of cooking time. Store in separate containers. Try using pre-shredded cabbage and pre-cut matchstick carrots.
2. Prepare the sauce ahead of time. Remix with a spoon when ready to heat. Use a spatula to remove the sauce to ensure that none is lost.

Nutrients Per Serving: 366 calories, 15 grams fat, 2 grams saturated fat, 20 grams protein, 42 grams carbohydrate, 7 grams fiber, 675 milligrams sodium

Lentillies

This flavorful and hearty sandwich is a plant-based version of a Whimpy or Sloppy Joe. A great side with this recipe is the easy Super Slaw recipe in this book. For variety, add a dollop of slaw on top of the Lentilly mix and either close the bun or keep it open-faced. Double the Lentilly recipe for leftovers that can be frozen easily for quick pull-out meals.

1 cup dried red lentils, rinsed	(190 grams)
2 cups (480 milliliters) water	(480 grams)
¾ cup diced (¼-inch sides) yellow or sweet onions	(120 grams)
¾ cup diced (¼-inch sides) green bell peppers	(110 grams)
8 ounces baby bella mushrooms, diced (¼-inch sides)	(230 grams)
15 ounces canned (400 milliliters) tomato sauce	(430 grams)
2 tablespoons (30 milliliters) unfiltered apple cider vinegar	(30 grams)
1 tablespoon granulated sugar	(10 grams)
2 teaspoons chili powder	(5 grams)
2 teaspoons plant beef flavor bouillon base or cubes for 2 cup equivalent, do not reconstitute	(10 grams)
1 teaspoon minced garlic	(3 grams)
2 tablespoons (30 milliliters) extra virgin olive oil	(25 grams)
8 hamburger style buns	(340 grams)
16 hamburger style dill chips	(60 grams)

Place lentils in a saucepan and cover with 2 cups of water. With the lid on, bring to a boil and turn down to a strong simmer for 5-6 minutes. Drain and set aside.

Place onions, bell peppers, mushrooms, tomato sauce, vinegar, sugar, chili powder, bouillon, and garlic in a large saucepan and mix by hand until well combined. Bring to a simmer with the lid on and cook for 10 minutes, stirring every 2 minutes to prevent sticking. Add lentils and olive oil, and continue to heat for 5 more minutes with the saucepan lid off.

Open buns and toast lightly on the inside. Use ⅔ cup Lentilly mixture and 2 pickle chips for each sandwich.

Servings: 8   **Serving size:** ⅔ cup of Lentilly mix and 1 bun, 2 pickle chips (170 grams)

Recommend with: Super Slaw, fresh fruit, and plant milk.

Notes:
1. To save time, consider cutting onions and bell peppers ahead of cooking time, and store in the refrigerator or freezer. Also, you can mix the tomato sauce, vinegar, sugar, chili powder, vinegar, bouillon, and garlic in a glass container ahead of cooking time, and store in the refrigerator.
2. Add ground turkey or chicken to individual servings for non-plant-based eaters.

Nutrients Per Serving: 270 calories, 6 grams fat, 1 grams saturated fat, 12 grams protein, 44 grams carbohydrate, 5 grams fiber, 765 milligrams sodium

Magnificent Macaroni Casserole

Children love the creamy inside and crunchy surface of this macaroni casserole. It is great when combined with Turnip Greens and Dumplings (recipe in this book) or just by itself!

Pasta

16 ounces (4¼ cups) dry whole-grain elbow pasta	(450 grams)
Cooking spray	

Toppings

¾ cup panko bread crumbs	(40 grams)
¾ cup shredded plant parmesan cheese	(80 grams)

Sauce

4 cups chopped cauliflower, from about ½ head	(400 grams)
2 cups (470 milliliters) water	(470 grams)
½ cup chopped carrots	(70 grams)
½ cup chopped yellow or sweet onions	(80 grams)
⅓ cup dried red lentils, rinsed	(65 grams)
¼ cup nutritional yeast	(20 grams)
1 teaspoon table salt	(6 grams)
¼ teaspoon black pepper	(1 gram)
½ teaspoon minced garlic	(1 gram)
½ cup plant butter	(110 grams)
1 cup (240 milliliters) unsweetened coconut milk refrigerated or boxed type, not canned, about 60 calories per cup	(230 grams)
2 tablespoons (30 milliliters) lemon juice	(30 grams)

For the pasta: In a large stockpot, boil 4 quarts of water. Add pasta and boil for 6 minutes or according to package directions. Drain and rinse pasta under cold water in a colander. Spray pasta with cooking spray and toss. Set aside.

For the toppings: Spread bread crumbs on a glass baking dish or sheet pan. Heat oven to 350°F (177°C). Place bread crumbs in the oven for about 10-15 minutes until golden brown. Set aside in a small bowl.

Set aside the parmesan cheese in a separate bowl.

For the sauce: Add the cauliflower, water, carrots, onions, lentils, yeast, salt, pepper, and garlic into a large stockpot. With the stockpot lid on, bring the ingredients to a boil and turn down to a simmer for 20 minutes. Remove from heat and allow to cool a bit. Puree with a hand blender until smooth. Add butter, coconut milk, and lemon juice. Stir until well combined. Reheat to a simmer or until warmed throughout.

To assemble: Add pasta to the sauce and stir until combined. Sprinkle bread crumbs and parmesan cheese over individual servings.

Servings: 10   **Serving size:** 1 cup pasta and sauce, 2 tablespoons topping (260 grams)

Recommend with: garden salad greens, fresh fruit, and plant milk.

Notes:
1. Double sauce and freeze half for later use. Thaw, reheat, and combine with freshly prepared noodles.
2. Add a side of shredded sharp cheddar cheese as a topping for non-plant-based eaters.

Nutrients Per Serving: 320 calories, 11 grams fat, 4 grams saturated fat, 11 grams protein, 48 grams carbohydrate, 6 grams fiber, 434 milligrams sodium

Night on the Mediterranean Gyro

Seasoned and grilled portabella mushroom tops help make this recipe so tasty. Adding my Tabouli Salad recipe and a protein rich plant milk increases the protein content of the meal. A broiler pan set or grill is needed to prepare this recipe, and parchment paper and aluminum foil are used to wrap the gyro.

Tzatziki sauce

¾ cup peeled and diced (¼-inch sides) English cucumber	(100 grams)
¼ teaspoon table salt, divided	(2 grams)
¾ cup plant sour cream	(170 grams)
⅛ teaspoon dried dill weed	(<1 gram)
1 teaspoon minced garlic	(3 grams)
2 tablespoons (30 milliliters) lemon juice	(30 grams)

Gyro

1½ cups torn (1-inch pieces) romaine lettuce	(70 grams)
1 cup halved grape or cherry tomatoes	(180 grams)
1 tablespoon (15 milliliters) balsamic vinegar	(15 grams)
1 tablespoon (15 milliliters) extra virgin olive oil	(15 grams)
¼ teaspoon table salt	(2 grams)
¼ teaspoon black pepper	(1 gram)
6 ounces large portobello mushroom tops, washed, dried, sliced lengthwise into thin strips	(170 grams)
Cooking spray	
4 pieces of flatbread	(10 grams)

Assembly preparation: Cut 4 rectangular (about 5 by 12 inches) sheets of aluminum foil and parchment paper, which are used to wrap and hold the gyro while eating. Set aside until assembly time.

For the tzatziki sauce: Place diced cucumber in a strainer with a bowl underneath. Sprinkle with ⅛ teaspoon salt and toss to distribute evenly. Allow the cucumber to sit in the strainer for 20 minutes. Rinse. Squeeze excess water from the cucumber with the back of a spoon and paper towels, and place cucumber in a bowl. Add sour cream, dill weed, and salt (⅛ teaspoon). If using pre-minced garlic, squeeze garlic with the back of a spoon to eliminate excess liquid. Add garlic and lemon juice to the mix and stir together. Place in the refrigerator to chill.

For the gyro: Prepare lettuce and tomatoes and set aside. Whisk together vinegar, oil, salt, and pepper in a medium-sized bowl. Wash, dry, and slice mushrooms tops, and coat with the vinegar oil mix. If using an oven, turn heat to broil. Spray the top of the broiler pan with cooking spray. Place mushrooms on top of the broiler pan set, about 6 inches from the oven's top heating element. Heat for 10 minutes on broil or until desired charring is present. A grill may be used instead.

To assemble: Cover aluminum foil with parchment paper and place a piece of flatbread on each. Distribute the lettuce and tomato evenly across the flatbread. Add mushroom slices and top with generous amounts of tzatziki sauce. Fold the bottom part of the flatbread one-third of the way up and then fold in the left and right sides to the middle. Secure by wrapping parchment paper and foil around the upper middle and bottom parts of the wrap.

Servings: 4 **Serving size:** 1 gyro (200 grams)

Recommend with: Tabouli Salad, fresh fruit, and plant milk.

Notes:
1. Try pre-minced garlic to save time.
2. Another side item that goes well with gyros are oven-baked potato wedges with plenty of extra virgin olive oil, salt, and garlic.
3. To satisfy non-plant-based eaters, consider making a side of browned ground turkey to be added individually.

Nutrients Per Serving: 448 calories, 19 grams fat, 5 grams saturated fat, 11 grams protein, 58 grams carbohydrate, 5 grams fiber, 840 milligrams sodium

Old Fashioned Squash Casserole

My dear grandmother, Mona, taught me how to make her delicious squash casserole. To increase the protein content of a meal featuring this plant-based version of her recipe, add a side of cooked fresh field peas.

½ cup plus 2 teaspoons dried navy beans or 15 ounces canned, drained	(110 grams)
2 pounds crookneck yellow squash, sliced (½-inch thick rounds) from about 6 medium squash	(910 grams)
1 cup chopped (½-inch sides) yellow or sweet onions	(160 grams)
1 cup plant sour cream	(220 grams)
2 teaspoons plant chicken flavor bouillon base or cubes for 2 cup equivalent, do not reconstitute	(10 grams)
¼ teaspoon table salt	(2 grams)
½ teaspoon black pepper	(1 grams)
8 ounces canned sliced water chestnuts, drained	(140 grams)
1 cup plant cheddar cheese	(110 grams)
Cooking spray	
¼ cup plant butter, softened not melted	(55 grams)
30 saltine or soda crackers, roughly broken	(100 grams)

Use the overnight or quick soaking method to prepare dried beans. Drain and then cover with plenty of fresh water. Bring to a boil and then turn down to a simmer for 1½-2 hours until tender. Remove from heat, drain, and cool. Refrigerate beans that you are not using right away.

Canned beans should be drained but not soaked or cooked.

Steam squash and onions in a large pot until tender (about 15 minutes). Do not overcook or the squash will be soggy. Drain water thoroughly. Chop squash a bit more.

Combine sour cream, bouillon, salt, and pepper in a large mixing bowl. Add the navy beans. Use an immersion blender to puree the bean mixture.

Add squash and onions to the bean puree. Fold in the water chestnuts and cheese until all ingredients are evenly distributed.

Spray a 9 x 13-inch glass baking dish with cooking spray. Evenly spread the squash casserole mixture in the baking dish. Heat uncovered on 375°F (190°C) for 30 minutes.

While the casserole is cooking, spread softened butter directly on saltine or soda crackers, and break crackers into several pieces in a separate baking dish. Place crackers in the oven with the casserole until crackers are golden brown (about 15 minutes). Use crackers as a spoon-on topping for individual servings of casserole.

Servings: 8 **Serving size:** ¾ cup squash (180 grams) and ¼ cup cracker topping (15 grams)

Recommend with: fresh field peas, fresh fruit, and plant milk.

Notes:
1. Soak and cook beans ahead of time and store in the refrigerator.
2. Chop onions ahead of cooking time and store in the refrigerator.
3. Add diced baked chicken breast to individual servings for non-plant-based eaters.

Nutrients Per Serving: 306 calories, 14 grams fat, 5 grams saturated fat, 7 grams protein, 41 grams carbohydrate, 6 grams fiber, 697 milligrams sodium

Red and White Pizzas

This recipe will create two delicious pizzas: one red/Basil Parmesan Pizza and one white/Artichoke Spinach Pizza. Try dipping cooked pizza in hummus, pesto, or pizza sauce for variety.

Dough (for two, 14-inch pizzas)

2½ cups (590 milliliters) warm water, not hot	(590 grams)
2 tablespoons and ¾ teaspoon active dry yeast or three, ¼ ounce, packets active yeast	(25 grams)
5¼ cups bread flour	(720 grams)
1½ teaspoons table salt	(9 grams)
2 tablespoons (30 milliliters) extra virgin olive oil	(25 grams)
Cooking spray	

Dough toppings (for two, 14-inch pizzas)

2 tablespoons plant butter, melted	(30 grams)
4 teaspoons nutritional yeast seasoning	(7 grams)
¼ teaspoon table salt	(2 grams)
1 teaspoon dried oregano or 1 tablespoon chopped fresh oregano	(4 grams)
2 teaspoons minced garlic	(10 grams)

Red pizza toppings

1 cup pizza sauce, divided	(250 grams)
½ cup shredded plant parmesan cheese	(60 grams)
1 cup fresh basil leaves	(25 grams)

White pizza toppings

1 cup marinated artichoke hearts, drained and sliced lengthways for thinner strips	(130 grams)
Cooking spray	
2.5 ounces (about 5 cups) fresh baby spinach	(70 grams)

For the dough: Heat water in a microwave oven for 1 minute to bring it to a warm but not hot temperature. Add yeast to the water, stir briefly, and let sit for 10 minutes.

Add bread flour and salt to a large mixing bowl. Mix together. Remove ¼ cup of the flour mixture and spread onto a work surface such as a large cutting board.

After 10 minutes, add the yeast mixture to the flour in the large mixing bowl. Stir the flour and yeast mixture with a large spoon until it is roughly mixed (about 20 stirs), scraping the sides of the bowl to push the mix into the center. Form the flour and yeast mixture into a loose dough ball with your hands. Place the dough ball on the floured cutting board or surface. Add the flour from the work surface to the dough, little by little, as you gently press down on the dough ball, and fold it over on itself about 7-10 times while retaining its spherical configuration.

Wash and dry the large mixing bowl. Coat the bowl interior with 2 tablespoons of extra virgin olive oil. Place the dough in the bowl and roll it around in the olive oil. Cover the bowl with a thin damp dish towel (flour sack towels work well) and set in a warm area for 1 hour or more to let the dough rise. Once the dough has risen, divide it into two equal portions.

Spray two, 14-inch pizza pans with cooking spray. Place the dough in the center of the pan. Using your hands, flatten and spread the dough out to the edge of the pan making it thinner in the center and thicker at the edges of the pan and being careful not to tear or overwork the dough. Drip the remaining olive oil from the bowl evenly onto the dough.

For the dough toppings: Place butter in a microwave safe dish and cover it with a paper towel. Microwave for about 20 seconds to melt. In a small bowl, combine nutritional yeast and salt with melted butter. Using a silicone pastry brush, lightly spread butter yeast mixture onto the dough in the pizza pans. Brush to cover the edges. Sprinkle oregano and garlic evenly over the dough.

For the red pizza toppings: Using a tablespoon, dot the red pizza dough with ¾ cup pizza sauce in evenly spaced dots. Use the back of a spoon to spread about slightly. Reserve ¼ cup pizza sauce in a bowl for dipping sauce while eating. Evenly spread the parmesan cheese and basil leaves on top of the pizza.

For the white pizza toppings: Evenly space the sliced artichoke hearts on the white pizza dough. Spray a saute pan with cooking spray. Cook spinach on medium-high until just wilted. Sprinkle a pinch of salt over spinach. Use a fork and knife to cut the spinach into smaller bite-size pieces and spread evenly on white pizza.

Bake each pizza separately at 425°F (218°C) degrees for 15-17 minutes. Use ¼ cup red pizza sauce for dipping as desired.

Servings: 8 (makes two, 14-inch pizzas-16 slices)   **Serving size:** two, ⅛ slices of pizza (200 grams)

Recommend with: Spring Side Salad, fresh fruit, and plant milk.

Notes:
1. Freeze one dough portion for later use if one pizza is all that is needed. After dough has risen in the bowl, freeze it in a gallon size bag with a little cooking spray. Label and date the bag. When you intend to use the frozen dough, thaw it in the bag overnight in the refrigerator.
2. If preparation of the dough in the pan is completed hours ahead of cooking time, cover the dough with parchment paper and set in the refrigerator. If making two pizzas at once, stack the pans on top of each other ensuring the dough is covered with parchment paper. Take them apart carefully. Add the toppings when ready to cook.
3. One way to satisfy those who want a purely plant-based pizza and others who desire cheese, is to sprinkle a little cheese over half of each pizza. Mozzarella works well with this recipe.

Nutrients Per Serving: 455 calories, 12 grams fat, 3 grams saturated fat, 16 grams protein, 71 grams carbohydrate, 5 grams fiber, 696 milligrams sodium

Savory Spaghetti

This delicious and nutrient rich spaghetti is quick and easy to make. Just add the ingredients to a stockpot, and it is done! This recipe yields a lot and works great for quick, pull-out of the freezer meals. Make the amount of noodles needed for the number to be served at the meal.

Spaghetti sauce

½ cup plus 2 teaspoons dried black beans	(100 grams)
or 15 ounces canned, drained	
½ cup dried chickpeas	(100 grams)
or 15 ounces canned, drained	
½ cup dried common brown lentils, rinsed	(95 grams)
1 cup chopped (½-inch sides) green bell peppers	(150 grams)
1 cup chopped (½-inch sides) yellow or sweet onions	(160 grams)
8 ounces fresh mushrooms, quartered or diced	(230 grams)
24 ounces (710 milliliters) plant spaghetti sauce	(750 grams)
30 ounces canned diced tomatoes	(820 grams)
1 cup (240 milliliters) water	(240 grams)
2 teaspoons plant beef flavor bouillon base	(10 grams)
or cube for 2 cup equivalent, do not reconstitute	
¼ teaspoon table salt	(2 grams)

Noodles (make in the amount needed for each meal)

8 ounces dry whole-grain thin spaghetti noodles	(230 grams)
for a 4-serving meal	
Cooking spray	

Topping (make in the amount needed for each meal)

¼ cup shredded plant parmesan cheese	(30 grams)
for a 4-serving meal	

For the beans: For dried black beans and dried chickpeas, use the overnight soak method. Soak black beans and chickpeas in separate pots, since black beans may discolor the chickpeas. Drain. In separate pots, cover the black beans and chickpeas with plenty of fresh water. Bring to a boil and then turn down to a simmer for 45 minutes. Drain and set aside.

Canned beans do not need additional preparation.

For the spaghetti sauce: Add black beans, chickpeas, lentils, bell peppers, onions, mushrooms, spaghetti sauce, tomatoes, water, bouillon, and salt to a large stockpot. Bring to a boil and then turn down to a simmer. Simmer covered for 45 minutes, stirring occasionally.

For the noodles: In another large stockpot, add about 8 cups of water and bring to a boil. Add the amount of noodles needed for the number of persons being served at that meal (2 ounces or 55 grams dry weight per person). Turn down to a simmer and cook for 6-7 minutes, or cook to al dente as directed on the package. Remove noodles from heat and drain in a colander. Run cold water over the noodles, drain and spray with cooking spray to prevent the noodles from sticking together.

Divide noodles among four serving bowls, and add spaghetti sauce on top. Sprinkle with plant parmesan cheese.

Servings: 11 cups sauce   **Serving size:** ¾ cup noodles (120 grams cooked), 1 cup sauce plus 1 tablespoon parmesan (250 grams)

Recommend with: Spring Side Salad, fresh fruit, plant garlic bread, and plant milk.

Notes:
1. Try slicing the vegetables into larger chunks for mature eaters and smaller pieces for those just starting out.
2. Once spaghetti sauce has cooled, scoop out enough for the current meal. Freeze the remaining spaghetti in family or individual meal-sized servings for future meals.
3. Penne pasta can also be used instead of spaghetti pasta for variety.
4. Add a small amount of ground turkey to individual servings to please non-plant-based eaters.

Nutrients Per Serving: 408 calories, 5 grams fat, 2 grams saturated fat, 17 grams protein, 78 grams carbohydrate, 14 grams fiber, 657 milligrams sodium

Sesame Garlic Vegetables and Tofu with Rice

Broccoli, red bell peppers, and sweet onions make a great mix of vegetables in this recipe, but many other vegetable combinations will also work well. Those who prefer a lot of sauce may wish to double the sauce ingredients. For another twist, try 1 tablespoon of molasses in place of sugar.

Tofu

14 ounces drained firm tofu block	(400 grams)
1 tablespoon (15 milliliters) canola oil	(15 grams)
1 tablespoon cornstarch	(8 grams)
Cooking spray	

Rice

2 cups (470 milliliters) water	(470 grams)
1 cup dry brown rice	(190 grams)

Sauce

¼ cup (60 milliliters) less sodium soy sauce	(60 grams)
2 tablespoons (30 milliliters) seasoned rice vinegar	(30 grams)
1 tablespoon plus 1 teaspoon granulated sugar	(15 grams)
1 teaspoon minced garlic	(3 grams)
1 teaspoon cornstarch	(3 grams)
2 tablespoons (30 milliliters) water	(30 grams)
2 teaspoons (10 milliliters) sesame oil	(10 grams)

Vegetables

3 cups cut (1-inch pieces) fresh broccoli florets	(270 grams)
1 cup chopped (½ or ¾-inch sides) yellow or sweet onions	(160 grams)
½ cup chopped (½ or ¾-inch sides) red bell peppers	(70 grams)

For the tofu: Begin preparing tofu 1-4 hours ahead of cooking time. Unwrap tofu and drain the liquid. Place tofu on a surface for cutting. Use a long, smooth, sharp knife to cut the tofu horizontally into two equal pieces that look like two slices of bread in a sandwich. Wrap both pieces completely with paper towels. Next, wrap the tofu (already in paper towels) with a thin, clean and dry dish towel. Place the wrapped tofu on a plate, and place another plate on top of the tofu with sufficient weight to compress the tofu and drain excess moisture. Refrigerate while compressing for 30 minutes. Replace the towels with fresh paper and cloth, and compress for another 20 minutes in the refrigerator.

For the rice: Refer to cooking instructions on the package. Add water to a 3-quart saucepan and bring to a boil. Add rice, cover with lid, and reduce temperature to medium-low to simmer rice for about 45 minutes or according to package directions. Remove from heat and keep covered.

For the sauce: Combine soy sauce, vinegar, sugar, and garlic in a bowl. Combine the cornstarch and water in a separate small bowl and stir until the cornstarch is dissolved. Mix the cornstarch and water in with the previous sauce ingredients. Place in a covered saucepan. Bring the sauce to a boil and quickly reduce to a simmer. Stir frequently until sauce has thickened a little, then remove from heat. Add sesame oil.

For the vegetables: Using a steamer basket and a 3-quart saucepan or stockpot, add 1-inch of water, and bring to a boil. Add broccoli and cover with a lid. Steam for about 4-5 minutes until the broccoli is cooked al dente (just tender but not mushy). Take off the heat and remove the lid. Spray a small saute pan with cooking spray. Heat the pan to medium-high. Add the bell peppers and onions and continue to heat for 5 minutes. Remove from heat and set aside.

For the tofu: Take tofu out of the refrigerator and carefully remove all wrappings. Combine canola oil and cornstarch to make a paste. Spread the paste evenly over all surfaces of the tofu (a silicone pastry brush works well for this task). Save the remaining cornstarch and oil paste for later use. Spray cooking spray on a large saute or fry pan and heat to medium or medium-high heat. Once the pan is hot, add both pieces of tofu side-by-side. Heat for 5 minutes or until tofu begins to turn golden. Carefully flip to the other side for 5 minutes or until tofu starts to turn golden. Now turn the tofu pieces together on each of their four sides and cook each side for a few minutes until golden. Take the tofu out of the pan onto a cutting board. Using a serrated knife, cut both pieces lengthwise. Brush the newly cut surfaces with the cornstarch and oil paste. Place all pieces in the pan on the side that hasn't been cooked for a minute or until golden. Place tofu back on the cutting board, and cut the tofu into 1-inch pieces. Brush the cornstarch and oil paste on the newly cut areas and heat those surfaces. Remove the pan from heat, but leave the tofu in the pan until ready to serve. Don't let it sit too long to avoid having it become chewy.

Serve on plates with a bed of rice under the broccoli mix with the tofu squares and a final drizzle of sauce on top.

Servings: 4 **Serving size:** ¾ cup rice, 1 cup vegetables, 3 pieces tofu, 2 tablespoons sauce **(370 grams)**

Recommend with: spring roll, fresh fruit, and plant milk.

Notes:
1. Mix the sauce ingredients together ahead of time and store in the refrigerator. Stir the cornstarch until it is dissolved again before heating.

Nutrients Per Serving: 449 calories, 16 grams fat, 2 grams saturated fat, 22 grams protein, 59 grams carbohydrate, 6 grams fiber, 691 milligrams sodium

Simple Leek Soup

This tasty soup is easy to prepare and inviting at any time of the year. The recipe makes enough for two suppers for a family of four.

1 cup plus 4 teaspoons dried navy beans	(210 grams)
or 30 ounces canned, drained	
4 cups sliced (¼-inch curls) leeks, divided, from about 2 leeks	(360 grams)
3 cups (710 milliliters) unsweetened coconut milk	(690 grams)
refrigerated or boxed type, not canned, about 60 calories per cup	
4 teaspoons plant chicken flavor bouillon base	(25 grams)
or cubes for 4 cup equivalent, do not reconstitute	
2 cups gold potato chunks (¾-inch sides) with skin	(350 grams)
½ cup plant butter	(110 grams)
1 tablespoon (15 milliliters) lemon juice	(15 grams)
8 sprigs parsley for garnish (optional)	(8 grams)

For the dried navy beans, use the overnight or quick soaking method to prepare the beans. Drain and then cover the beans with plenty of fresh water. Bring to a boil and turn down to a simmer for 1½-2 hours until beans are tender. Remove from heat, drain, and cool. Refrigerate beans that you are not using right away.

Canned beans should be drained but not soaked or cooked.

Using kitchen shears, remove the dark green parts of the leek leaves and discard. Keep the lighter green stalk. Section the leek stalk into quarters keeping the root end intact by using a large sharp knife or chef knife to make a lengthwise slice starting ½-inch from the root end and continuing to the opposite end. Quarter turn the stalk and make another similar slice. Now the leek is sectioned in quarters but still intact at the root. Thoroughly wash the leek with water until all dirt is removed. Hold the root end lengthwise and starting at the opposite end of the root, make ¼-inch slices creating round or curl shaped pieces. When you are about ¼-½ inch from the root end, stop slicing and discard the root end. Boil the leek pieces in water for 15 minutes and drain. Set aside.

Combine the beans, leeks, coconut milk, and bouillon in a bowl, and use an immersion or standard blender to puree until smooth. A spatula helps to remove all puree from the bowl or blender.

Add the bean and leek puree, potatoes and butter to a 6-quart or larger stockpot. Heat to a simmer (covered) and cook for 15-18 minutes, stirring frequently to prevent sticking on the bottom. Avoid overcooking to keep potatoes intact. Add lemon juice to the soup when cooking is complete.

Serve in bowls and garnish with a sprig of parsley.

Servings: 8   **Serving size:** 1 cup (250 grams)

Recommend with: whole-grain bread, fresh fruit, and plant milk.

Notes:
1. Watch a how-to video from the internet to observe how to cut a leek.
2. Wash and chop leeks ahead of time and store in the refrigerator.
3. Sprinkle shredded plant cheddar on top of any serving. Consider regular shredded cheddar for non-plant-based eaters.

Nutrients Per Serving: 259 calories, 11 grams fat, 4 grams saturated fat, 7 grams protein, 32 grams carbohydrate, 9 grams fiber, 434 milligrams sodium

Southern Black-eyed Peas

Black-eyed peas are enjoyed by people all over the world. They are a good source of protein, fiber, and iron. Ripe tomato slices and a piece of cornbread make delicious sides. In addition, the tomatoes (depending on the variety) provide vitamin C which helps your body absorb the iron from the peas.

2 cups (12 ounces) dried black-eyed peas	(340 grams)
4½ cups (1,070 milliliters) water	(1,070 grams)
3 cups chopped (½-inch sides) yellow or sweet onions	(480 grams)
2 tablespoons (30 milliliters) less sodium soy sauce	(30 grams)
1 tablespoon plant chicken flavor bouillon base or cubes for 3 cup equivalent, do not reconstitute	(20 grams)

Prepare dried black-eyed peas ahead of time by soaking the peas for 8 hours or overnight. Place peas in a large stockpot (6-quart or larger). Immerse peas completely in water and cover with the stockpot lid while soaking.

After soaking, drain and add fresh water (4½ cups). Add the remaining ingredients. Bring to a boil. Once boiling turn down to a simmer (covered) for 1 hour to 1 hour and 10 minutes. Peas should be soft but not mushy. Overcooked peas become mushy, so begin checking at 1 hour for desired softness.

Servings: 8   **Serving size:** 1 cup (240 grams)

Recommend with: tomato slices, Meltaway Cornbread, fresh fruit, and plant milk.

Notes:
1. Onions may be cut ahead of cooking time and stored in the refrigerator or freezer.
2. The onions, soy sauce, and bouillon may be added while the peas are heating or within the first 10 minutes of simmering to shorten preparation time.

Nutrients Per Serving: 150 calories, 1 gram fat, 0 grams saturated fat, 9 grams protein, 33 grams carbohydrate, 8 grams fiber, 398 milligrams sodium

Spiced Beanloaf

This plant-based version of meatloaf is great with my Parsley Mashed Potatoes and Buttered Sweet Peas recipes.

½ cup plus 2 teaspoons dried black beans or 15 ounces canned, drained	(100 grams)
½ cup dried chickpeas or 15 ounces canned, drained	(100 grams)
½ cup dried red lentils, rinsed	(95 grams)
2 cups (470 milliliters) water	(470 grams)
1 cup peeled and diced (¼-inch sides) celery lightly peel tough outer layer	(140 grams)
1 cup diced (¼-inch sides) yellow or sweet onions	(160 grams)
½ cup diced (¼-inch sides) bell peppers	(80 grams)
Cooking spray	
1 tablespoon (15 milliliters) apple cider vinegar	(15 grams)
1 tablespoon minced garlic (see Note 2)	(9 grams)
1 tablespoon plant beef flavor bouillon base or cube for 3 cup equivalent, do not reconstitute	(20 grams)
1 teaspoon (5 milliliters) less sodium soy sauce	(5 grams)
½ teaspoon ground cumin	(1 gram)
½ teaspoon ground nutmeg	(1 gram)
½ teaspoon table salt	(3 grams)
¼ teaspoon ground red pepper	(<1 gram)
2 tablespoons (30 milliliters) extra virgin olive oil	(25 grams)
½ cup ketchup	(120 grams)
¼ cup 5-minute quick grits	(40 grams)
½ cup (120 milliliters) unsweetened soymilk	(120 grams)
3 tablespoons ground flaxseed	(20 grams)
¾ cup panko bread crumbs	(40 grams)

Use the overnight or quick soaking method to prepare the dried black beans and dried chickpeas. Soak the beans and peas separately since black beans may discolor the chickpeas. Drain. In separate pots cover black beans and chickpeas with plenty of fresh water. Bring each pot to a boil and then turn down to a strong simmer for about 1-1½ hours until beans and peas are tender. Remove from heat, drain, and cool. Refrigerate black beans and chickpeas that you are not using right away.

Canned black beans and chickpeas should be drained but not soaked or cooked.

Add lentils and 2 cups water to a saucepan. Heat to boiling and boil for exactly 5 minutes. Drain.

Dice the celery, onions, and peppers. Spray a large saute pan with cooking spray and add lentils, celery, onions, bell peppers, vinegar, garlic, bouillon, soy sauce, cumin, nutmeg, salt, and red pepper. Cook over medium heat (uncovered) for 10 minutes, stirring occasionally so vegetables do not stick. Reduce the temperature to medium-low. Combine olive oil, ketchup, and grits in a bowl and add to the lentil-vegetable mixture. Continue cooking for another 10 minutes, stirring occasionally. Then, stir in the soymilk, remove from heat, and allow to cool a bit.

Add black beans and chickpeas to a bowl, and use a potato masher to break them up into a rough mixture. Coat a 9 x 13-inch glass baking dish with cooking spray. In the baking dish, combine the black bean-chickpea mix with the lentil-vegetable mix. In a separate bowl, combine the flaxseed and panko bread crumbs, and add this to the beanloaf mixture in the baking dish. Using your hands, combine the ingredients thoroughly and shape the mixture into a loaf about 1-inch high in the center of the dish. Leave about ½ inch of space between the loaf and the sides of the baking dish.

Store in the refrigerator, covered, until time to bake. Cover the dish with aluminum foil and bake on 350°F (177°C) for 40 minutes. Remove foil, turn the heat to broil, and broil for 3 minutes. Remove from oven and allow beanloaf to sit for 10 minutes before serving.

Servings: 12 **Serving size:** 1/12 of loaf (110 grams)

Recommend with: Parsley Mashed Potatoes or rice, Buttered Sweet Peas or Sauteed Asparagus, fresh fruit, and plant milk.

Notes:
1. Dice vegetables ahead of time. Store extra vegetables in the freezer for future use. Be sure to label and date.
2. Try using a pre-minced garlic to save time.
3. Measure and combine ingredients ahead of cooking time. In one bowl add vinegar, garlic, bouillon, soy sauce, cumin, nutmeg, salt, and red pepper. Measure out flaxseed and panko bread crumbs to another bowl.

Nutrients Per Serving: 171 calories, 4 grams fat, 1 gram saturated fat, 8 grams protein, 27 grams carbohydrate, 6 grams fiber, 403 milligrams sodium

Spinach and Sweet Pepper Quiche

Serve this quiche with fresh fruit for a delicious combination. A spring mix side salad with your favorite dressing makes for the ultimate finishing touch.

Crust
1¼ cups all-purpose flour	(160 grams)
1 teaspoon granulated sugar	(4 grams)
¼ teaspoon table salt	(2 grams)
½ cup cold plant butter	(110 grams)
3 tablespoons (45 milliliters) ice water	(45 grams)
Cooking spray	

Filling
Cooking spray	
1 cup chopped (½-inch sides) yellow or sweet onions	(120 grams)
½ cup chopped (½-inch sides) red bell peppers	(60 grams)
5 ounces (about 10 cups) fresh baby spinach	(140 grams)
2 tablespoons unsweetened soymilk	(30 grams)
1 tablespoon ground flaxseed	(7 grams)
1 tablespoon minced garlic	(9 grams)
2 teaspoons plant chicken flavor bouillon base or cube for 2 cup equivalent, do not reconstitute	(10 grams)
¼ teaspoon table salt	(2 grams)
¼ teaspoon turmeric	(1 gram)
14 ounces drained firm tofu block	(400 grams)
¼ cup shredded plant parmesan cheese	(30 grams)

For the crust: Mix the flour, sugar, and salt together in a bowl. Remove 2 tablespoons of the dry mixture and set aside for a moment. Cut cold butter into the main mixture with a pastry cutter until the butter is reduced to small pea-sized pieces. Sprinkle the remaining 2 tablespoons of dry mixture over the pea-sized pieces. Stir the entire bowl by scooping and lifting the dough a few times with a fork. Sprinkle the dough with ice water, one tablespoon at a time, followed by a quick stir with a fork after each spoonful. Compress the mixture together gently with your hands to form a dough ball. Wrap the ball in parchment paper, secure with a tie, and place in the refrigerator to chill for 30 minutes or longer if working ahead.

When ready to prepare the pie shell, spray a 9-inch glass or ceramic pie pan with cooking spray. Take the dough from the refrigerator, unwrap the parchment and place the dough on the pan with the parchment paper above it. Press on the top side of the parchment paper with a small roller such as a 4-inch mini pizza dough roller or 6-inch mini French rolling pin (or with your hand in a pinch) to flatten and roll the dough onto the bottom of the pie pan. Roll from the middle outward so that the dough closer to the side of the pan is slightly thicker. Use your fingers to work the thicker outer dough ring up the side to the top of the pie pan. Leave the smooth or fluted edge of the pan free of dough. Prick the bottom of the pie crust with a fork in several places. Bake at 400°F (204°C) for 8 minutes.

Alternatively, use a pre-made pie crust. Follow package instructions for baking before adding quiche filling. Wrap the outer fluted edge of a pre-made pie crust with aluminum foil to prevent burning.

For the filling: Spray a large skillet or saute pan with cooking spray and heat to medium. Add onions and peppers, and use a spoon to push them around in the pan for about 10 minutes to allow water to cook out. Turn down the heat if the vegetables start to brown. Add spinach to the onions and peppers and cook for 5-6 additional minutes. Remove from heat, and use a fork and sharp knife to cut the spinach into smaller pieces. Set aside.

Place soymilk, flaxseed, garlic, bouillon, salt, and turmeric into a bowl and mix together with a fork. Drain tofu and add to the bowl. Use a hand blender to integrate the tofu with the other ingredients. Mix until fully combined. Use a silicone spoon spatula to remove and combine all the tofu mixture with the spinach mixture. Add the combined mixture evenly within the pie crust, and spread the filling with a spatula to cover the crust up to the top edge on the side of the pan but not the fluted edge if using a pre-made crust. Smooth the top of the quiche filling with the back of the spatula. Sprinkle the shredded parmesan on top.

Bake at 400°F (204°C) for 60 minutes. Check the middle of the quiche for doneness by inserting a knife in and peeking to see if the quiche has congealed to a soft-formed stage. If it still has a wet/liquid look to it, continue baking for another 20-30 minutes until done. Allow to sit for 5 minutes before serving.

Servings: 8   **Serving size:** ⅛ of quiche (130 grams)

Recommend with: Spring Side Salad, fresh fruit, and plant milk.

Notes:
1. Chop vegetables and make the dough ball ahead of cooking time. Store in the refrigerator.
2. Double pie crust recipe. Wrap the additional pie crust dough ball in parchment paper, and freeze in a labeled and dated plastic bag. Allow to thaw overnight in the refrigerator before using.
3. Double recipe and freeze one quiche. Work through the steps of baking the crust and adding filling in the shell. Carefully, place the uncooked quiche in the freezer uncovered. Once it freezes and within a few hours, remove from the freezer and cover well with plastic wrap and a gallon size bag if the pie pan will fit. Label and date and return to freezer. Do not allow the quiche to thaw before cooking. Wrap the edge with a narrow ring of aluminum foil to prevent burning. Lay a square sheet of aluminum foil on top of the quiche to fully cover it, but do not wrap it closed. Bake at 400°F (204°C) for 60 minutes. Remove the square sheet of foil and continue baking for another 30 minutes.
4. Consider sprinkling additional favorite shredded cheese over half of the quiche during the last 5 minutes of cooking to please non-plant-based eaters.

Nutrients Per Serving: 226 calories, 13 grams fat, 3 grams saturated fat, 7 grams protein, 21 grams carbohydrate, 2 grams fiber, 459 milligrams sodium

Split Pea and Carrot Soup

What goes together better than peas and carrots? Split Pea Soup is one of the healthiest dishes, given all the protein, fiber, antioxidants, and other phytonutrients it provides. It is also one of the easiest to make!

6 cups (1,420 milliliters) of water	(1,420 grams)
1 tablespoon plant chicken flavor bouillon base or cubes for 3 cup equivalent, do not reconstitute	(20 grams)
1 cup sliced (¼-inch thick rounds) carrots	(130 grams)
1 cup chopped (½-inch sides) yellow or sweet onions	(160 grams)
⅛ teaspoon table salt	(1 gram)
2¼ cups (16 ounces) dried green split peas	(450 grams)

Add water, bouillon base, carrots, onions, and salt to a 6-quart stockpot and bring to a boil. Rinse and sort the split peas to remove any foreign materials or bad peas. Add peas to the stockpot as soon as the water boils. Cover and turn down to a simmer for 30 minutes. Avoid overcooking.

Servings: 9   **Serving size:** 1 cup (240 grams)

Recommend with: whole-grain roll, fresh fruit, and plant milk.

Notes:
1. Chop onions ahead of time to keep in the freezer and pull out when needed.
2. Cut the carrots ahead of time and keep them in the refrigerator. For convenience, use pre-washed baby carrots to cut into rounds.
3. Store leftover split peas in the refrigerator for the next evening's meal or freeze (label and date).
4. To please non-plant-based eaters, add a small serving of ham steak pieces to individual servings.

Nutrients Per Serving: 190 calories, 1 gram fat, 0 grams saturated fat, 13 grams protein, 34 grams carbohydrate, 14 grams fiber, 271 milligrams sodium

Tasty Tacos

Tacos are an easy meal to make. Many of the ingredients can be prepared ahead of cooking time to move the mealtime process along faster. Also, children can learn to help with such preparations as washing and breaking the lettuce into smaller pieces. For a crowd pleaser, this recipe can be easily doubled or tripled.

½ cup plus 2 teaspoons dried black beans	(100 grams)
or 15 ounces canned	
½ cup plus 2 teaspoons dried pinto beans	(100 grams)
or 15 ounces canned	
¼ teaspoon table salt, divided	(2 grams)
½ cup water	(120 grams)
Cooking spray	
1 cup frozen cut yellow corn	(160 grams)
2 cups shredded (½-inch pieces) lettuce	(90 grams)
2 cups halved cherry tomatoes	(360 grams)
½ cup chopped fresh cilantro	(8 grams)
½ cup sliced (¼-inch thick rounds) scallions	(50 grams)
1 cup prepared salsa	(260 grams)
½ cup plant sour cream	(110 grams)
8 large (6 ounces) hard taco shells	(160 grams)
1 medium Hass avocado, quartered and peeled	(140 grams)

For dried black and dried pinto beans, use the overnight soaking method to prepare the beans. Soak the beans separately since black beans may discolor pinto beans. Drain. In separate pots cover the beans with plenty of fresh water. Bring each to a boil and then turn down to a strong simmer for about 45 minutes to 1 hour for the black beans and 1½ hours for the pinto beans until the beans are tender. Drain.

For canned black and pinto beans, boil for 5 minutes in separate pots. Drain and set aside in separate containers.

Season black beans with ⅛ teaspoon salt and set aside. Add ⅛ teaspoon salt and ½ cup water to pinto beans and mash with a potato masher or hand blender to a lumpy smooth consistency. Set aside. Canned beans often have salt already added and may not need more.

Spray a saute pan with cooking spray and heat to medium. Add corn and cook until the corn has caramelized some, about 10 minutes. Remove from heat and set aside.

Prepare lettuce, tomatoes, cilantro, and scallions, and refrigerate in separate covered serving bowls until time to serve. Place salsa and sour cream in separate serving bowls.

Using a paring knife, slice the avocado lengthwise into quarters, hitting the seed with each slice. Use the knife as a wedge between slices to release the pieces. Remove and discard the seed and outer skin. Slice avocado quarters into smaller pieces if you prefer.

Heat oven to 325°F (163°C), place taco shells on a sheet pan and bake for 6-7 minutes. Follow the package directions.

Stuff tacos with pinto beans, lettuce, tomatoes, corn, cilantro, scallions, and salsa. Add avocados and a tablespoon of sour cream on top.

Serve black beans with a dollop of sour cream as a side to each plate.

Servings: 4   **Serving size:** ¼ of all ingredients, 2 tacos (490 grams)

Recommend with: fresh fruit and plant milk.

Notes:
1. Shred lettuce ahead of time. Romaine or green leaf lettuce works well.
2. Cut tomatoes, cilantro, and scallions ahead of time and store in separate bowls for serving. Also, place salsa and sour cream into small separate serving bowls with a cover ahead of cooking time so you can just pull them out when getting ready for the meal.
3. Watch a how-to video from the internet on how to cut avocados as needed.
4. For non-plant-based eaters, include a small side of seasoned ground turkey and shredded cheese.

Nutrients Per Serving: 583 calories, 20 grams fat, 6 grams saturated fat, 20 grams protein, 86 grams carbohydrate, 19 grams fiber, 937 milligrams sodium

Topside Pot Pie

This unconventional warm pot pie is a comfort food for all seasons. Serve with a chilled spring mix salad and fresh fruit to create a great balance of warm, cold, soft, crunchy, salty and sweet sensations in a colorful, nutrient-rich meal.

Crust

1¼ cups all-purpose flour	(160 grams)
1 teaspoon granulated sugar	(4 grams)
¼ teaspoon table salt	(2 grams)
½ cup cold plant butter	(110 grams)
3 tablespoons (45 milliliters) ice water	(45 grams)
Cooking spray	

Filling

1 cup plus 2 teaspoons dried navy beans or 30 ounces canned, drained	(220 grams)
1 cup (240 milliliters) water	(240 grams)
1 cup sliced (¼-inch thick rounds) carrots	(130 grams)
1 cup peeled and chopped (½-inch sides) celery lightly peel tough outer layer	(100 grams)
2 cups potato chunks (¾-inch sides) with skin from about 2 potatoes, 2 by 4 inches each	(350 grams)
4 teaspoons plant chicken flavor bouillon base or cubes for 4 cup equivalent, do not reconstitute	(25 grams)
½ teaspoon table salt	(3 grams)
¼ teaspoon black pepper	(1 gram)
¼ teaspoon dried thyme	(<1 gram)
2 cups (470 milliliters) unsweetened coconut milk, divided refrigerated or boxed type, not canned, about 60 calories per cup	(460 grams)
1 cup frozen green peas	(140 grams)

For the beans: For dried navy beans, use the overnight or quick soaking method to prepare the beans. Drain and then cover the beans with plenty of fresh water. Bring to a boil and then turn down to a strong simmer for 1½ hours until the beans are tender. Drain and set aside. When cool, place beans in the refrigerator if you are not using them right away.

Canned navy beans do not require preliminary soaking and cooking. Open can and drain when ready to puree (see Note 4).

For the crust: Mix flour, sugar, and salt together in a bowl. Remove 2 tablespoons of the dry mixture and set aside for a moment. Cut cold butter into the main dough mixture with a pastry cutter until it resembles small pea-sized pieces. Sprinkle the remaining 2 tablespoons of dry mixture over the pea-sized pieces. Stir the entire bowl by scooping and lifting the dough ingredients a few times with a fork. Sprinkle the dough with ice water, one tablespoon at a time, followed by a quick stir with the fork after each tablespoon. Compress the mixture gently with your hands to form a dough ball. Wrap the ball in parchment paper, secure with a tie, and place in the refrigerator to chill for 30 minutes or longer if working ahead.

When you are ready to bake the crust, spray a 9 x 13-inch glass baking dish with cooking spray. Remove the dough from the refrigerator, unwrap the parchment and place the dough on the pan with the parchment paper above it. Press on the top side of the parchment paper to flatten and roll the dough ball onto the bottom of the baking dish (not up the sides). First, use your hands to flatten the dough ball, then follow with a small roller, such as a 4-inch mini pizza dough roller or 6-inch mini French rolling pin (or continue to press with your hands in a pinch). Be sure to roll and press the dough evenly over the entire bottom of the baking dish. With a sharp knife, slice the dough into 8 equal rectangles. Bake on 400°F (204°C) for 20 minutes. Use a metal spatula to lift the crust squares when ready to serve.

For the filling: Puree beans with 1 cup water in a blender until silky smooth and pour into a saucepan. Use a rubber spatula to remove all the bean mixture from the blender. Add the carrots, celery, potato, bouillon, salt, pepper, and thyme to the saucepan. Add 1 cup of coconut milk. Cover and bring to a simmer for 18 minutes. Stir frequently to prevent food sticking to the bottom of the pan. Add the remaining 1 cup of coconut milk and the green peas. Cover and bring back to a simmer for 2 more minutes.

Scoop 1 cup of the filling into each bowl. Set 1 square to the side of the filling.

Servings: 8   **Serving size:** 1 cup of filling and 1 crust piece (280 grams)

Recommend with: garden salad greens, fresh fruit, and plant milk.

Notes:
1. Prepare all the vegetables, except the potato, ahead of cooking time and store in the refrigerator.

2. Use baby carrots to save time. Line them side-by-side like logs, and use a long knife to cut them.
3. Prepare dough ahead of time and store in the refrigerator.
4. Use canned beans to save time. Two, 15 ounces each, cans of beans yields 3 cups of cooked beans. Drain cans and puree with 1 cup water per recipe instructions.
5. To please non-plant-based eaters, cook a single chicken breast and pull apart into small pieces to add to individual servings.

Nutrients Per Serving: 328 calories, 11 grams fat, 4 grams saturated fat, 10 grams protein, 47 grams carbohydrate, 10 grams fiber, 694 milligrams sodium

Turnip Greens and Dumplings

I remember picking Fall turnip greens with my mother when I was a little girl. Now you can purchase fresh turnip greens throughout the year.

Turnip greens

6 cups (1,420 milliliters) water	(1,420 grams)
1 tablespoon plant chicken flavor bouillon base or cubes for 3 cup equivalent, do not reconstitute	(20 grams)
2 teaspoons (10 milliliters) less sodium soy sauce	(10 grams)
¼ teaspoon table salt	(2 grams)
16 ounces (about 16 cups) fresh chopped turnip greens, divided	(450 grams)

Dumplings

2 tablespoons (30 milliliters) plant butter, melted	(30 grams)
1 tablespoon flaxseed flour	(7 grams)
¾ cup white cornmeal	(120 grams)
¼ cup 5-minute quick grits	(40 grams)
1 teaspoon baking powder	(5 grams)
⅛ teaspoon paprika	(<1 gram)
⅛ teaspoon table salt	(1 gram)
½ cup (120 milliliters) pot liquor (turnip green broth)	(120 grams)

For the turnip green pot liquor: Add water, bouillon base, soy sauce, and salt to a 6-quart or larger stockpot. Chop several turnip green leaves into very small pieces and add in the pot. Bring to a boil with the lid on and then turn heat to the lowest setting. Keep covered to avoid losing any liquid.

For the dumplings: Melt 2 tablespoons butter in a small bowl. Add flaxseed flour to the butter and set aside. Combine cornmeal, grits, baking powder, paprika, and salt in a medium-sized bowl and set aside. Add ½ cup of the warm pot liquor with turnip green pieces to the butter and flaxseed mixture. Next, add the combined pot liquor and flaxseed butter to the dry cornmeal mixture and stir until well combined. Let the dumpling mixture sit out for 10 minutes.

Add the remaining turnip greens to the remaining pot liquor in the stockpot. Scoop a heaping tablespoon of dumpling mixture and compress the mixture between the spoon and your hand to form a dumpling. Make 8 dumplings and place them carefully on top of the dry greens in the pot so that the dumplings do not touch each other. Dust any dumpling crumbles from the bowl or hands over the greens. Bring the greens to a simmer, cover, and heat on medium for 30 minutes.

Servings: 8 **Serving size:** 1 cup of greens with pot liquor and dumpling (240 grams)

Recommend with: fresh field peas, fresh fruit, and plant milk.

Notes:
1. Measure dry ingredients for dumplings ahead of time.
2. To please non-plant-based eaters, add a small serving of cooked ham steak pieces for individuals. Freeze remaining ham steak for a later meal.

Nutrients Per Serving: 123 calories, 3 grams fat, 1 gram saturated fat, 3 grams protein, 21 grams carbohydrate, 3 grams fiber, 494 milligrams sodium

Vegetable Divan

This warm and inviting dish has a hint of curry. Feed a family of 4 and still have leftovers for another supper. Make this dish more easily by preparing the sauce and cutting the vegetables in advance.

1 cup plus 2 teaspoons dried northern beans	(210 grams)
or 15 ounces canned, drained	
½ cup (120 milliliters) water	(120 grams)
⅛ teaspoon table salt	(1 gram)
8 ounces fresh mushrooms, diced	(230 grams)
1 cup peeled and chopped (½-inch sides) celery	(120 grams)
lightly peel tough outer layer	
1 cup chopped (½-inch sides) yellow or sweet onions	(160 grams)
6 cups cut fresh broccoli florets in 1-inch pieces	(550 grams)
Cooking spray	
1 tablespoon plant chicken flavor bouillon base	(20 grams)
or cubes for 3 cup equivalent, do not reconstitute	
1 teaspoon curry	(2 grams)
1 cup plant mayonnaise	(220 grams)
1 cup (240 milliliters) unsweetened coconut milk	(230 grams)
refrigerated or boxed type, not canned, about 60 calories per cup	
½ cup (120 milliliters) white cooking wine	(120 grams)
2 tablespoons (30 milliliters) lemon juice	(30 grams)

Topping

½ cup panko bread crumbs	(25 grams)
½ cup shredded plant parmesan cheese	(55 grams)

For dried northern beans, use the overnight or quick soaking method to prepare the beans. Drain and then cover the beans with plenty of fresh water. Bring to a boil and turn down to a simmer for 1½-2 hours until beans are tender. Remove from heat, drain, and cool. Refrigerate beans that you are not using right away.

Canned beans should be drained but not soaked or cooked.

Add ½ cup fresh water and salt to beans. Canned beans often have salt already added and may not need more. Using a blender, puree beans until smooth and set aside.

Dice mushrooms, and chop celery and onions. Set aside. Cut broccoli into florets and set aside.

Heat a stockpot to medium heat and spray with cooking spray. Add mushrooms, celery, and onions to the stockpot. Stir occasionally so the vegetables do not stick to the pot. Cook uncovered for about 10 minutes. Add the broccoli and cook for another 10 minutes covered, stirring once or twice to help all vegetables cook evenly. Remove vegetables from heat and set aside.

In a medium-sized mixing bowl, combine the bouillon, curry, mayonnaise, and ½ cup of coconut milk and whisk together until smooth. Whisk in the rest of the coconut milk. Stir in the cooking wine and lemon juice. Add the pureed beans to the mixture using a spatula to transfer all the puree.

Spray a 9 x 13-inch glass baking dish with cooking spray. Add the seasoned coconut milk and bean mixture to the baking dish. Next, add the vegetable mixture.

Place the uncovered baking dish in a 400°F (204°C) oven for 30 minutes or until heated throughout.

For the topping: While the Divan is cooking in the oven, evenly distribute the bread crumbs and parmesan cheese in a small pan, and place in the oven. Remove when bread crumbs are crispy brown (about 10-15 minutes).

Serve the Divan in a bowl topped with 2 tablespoons of breadcrumbs.

Servings: 8   **Serving size:** 1 cup Divan, 2 tablespoons topping (250 grams)

Recommend with: brown rice or whole-grain roll, fresh fruit, and plant milk.

Notes:
1. Chop all vegetables ahead of time.
2. Combine the bouillon, curry, mayonnaise, coconut milk, wine, and lemon juice ahead of time and store in a sealed container.
3. May cook a small amount of a chicken breast torn into small pieces to add to individual servings for non-plant-based eaters.

Nutrients Per Serving: 312 calories, 17 grams fat, 4 grams saturated fat, 9 grams protein, 33 grams carbohydrate, 7 grams fiber, 505 milligrams sodium

Side Recipes

Buttered Sweet Peas   140
Classic Hummus   141
Meltaway Cornbread   143
Parsley Mashed Potatoes   144
Sauteed Asparagus   146
Seasonal Fresh Fruit Medley   147
Spring Side Salad   148
Super Slaw   150
Tabouli Salad   151

Buttered Sweet Peas

Sweet green peas are legumes that are full of protein, fiber, vitamins, minerals, antioxidants, and other phytonutrients known to support health. These hard-working peas make a colorful splash to any meal and are easy to keep on hand in the freezer. Even better, they only take minutes to prepare.

¼ cup (60 milliliters) water	(60 grams)
2 cups frozen green peas	(290 grams)
1 tablespoon plant butter	(15 grams)
⅛ teaspoon table salt	(1 gram)

Add water to a 2-quart saucepan and bring to a boil. Add peas. Cook for 2 minutes. Remove from heat and drain. Return peas to the pan or serving bowl, and add butter and salt. Stir until combined.

Servings: 4   **Serving size:** ½ cup (75 grams)

Recommend with: Spiced Beanloaf, Parsley Mashed Potatoes, or any meal.

Nutrients Per Serving: 76 calories, 3 grams fat, 1 gram saturated fat, 4 grams protein, 10 grams carbohydrate, 3 grams fiber, 174 milligrams sodium

Classic Hummus

Offer your family this hummus for a snack or appetizer and watch it disappear. Hummus is a good source of fiber which promotes a healthy intestinal microbiome. It also contains 6 grams of protein per serving which helps to meet daily protein needs.

½ cup dried chickpeas or 15 ounces canned	(100 grams)
2 tablespoons (30 milliliters) water	(30 grams)
2 tablespoons (30 milliliters) extra virgin olive oil	(25 grams)
1 tablespoon plus 1 teaspoon (20 milliliters) lemon juice	(20 grams)
1 tablespoon tahini paste	(15 grams)
½ teaspoon ground cumin	(1 gram)
½ teaspoon minced garlic	(1 gram)
½ teaspoon table salt	(3 grams)

Prepare dried chickpeas by using the overnight or quick soak method. Drain and then cover with plenty of fresh water. Bring to a boil and then turn down to a simmer for 1½-2 hours. Drain well and set aside.

Boil canned chickpeas with liquid from the can in a saucepan for 5-10 minutes. Remove from heat, drain and set aside to cool.

Add the water, olive oil, lemon juice, tahini, cumin, garlic, and salt to a medium-sized bowl and mix together. Add chickpeas to the mixed ingredients. Puree into a thick smooth consistency with an immersion blender. Use a spatula to gather all ingredients. Refrigerate until serving time.

Servings: 4 (makes 1¼ cups)   **Serving size:** 5 tablespoons (75 grams)

Recommend with: Crisp Vegetables and Hummus Sandwich, vegetables, or whole-grain pita pieces.

Notes:
1. May use a total of up to 3 tablespoons water as needed or desired.
2. Reduce salt by ⅛ teaspoon (25%) if too salty for your taste.
3. Try using pre-minced garlic to save time.

Nutrients Per Serving: 185 calories, 10 grams fat, 1 gram saturated fat, 6 grams protein, 18 grams carbohydrate, 5 grams fiber, 304 milligrams sodium

Meltaway Cornbread

This cornbread is smooth and has a melt-in-your-mouth feel. Give it a hint of sweetness by adding a tablespoon of sugar if you like.

1¼ cups white cornmeal	(200 grams)
¾ cup all-purpose flour	(90 grams)
2 tablespoons ground flaxseed	(15 grams)
1 tablespoon baking powder	(15 grams)
¼ teaspoon table salt	(2 grams)
1 cup (240 milliliters) unsweetened coconut milk refrigerated or boxed type, not canned, about 60 calories per cup	(240 grams)
¼ cup (120 milliliters) canola oil	(110 grams)
1 tablespoon (15 milliliters) white vinegar	(15 grams)
½ cup (120 milliliters) unsweetened applesauce	(120 grams)
¼ cup small-grated carrots	(30 grams)
Cooking spray	

Combine dry ingredients (cornmeal, flour, flaxseed, baking powder, and salt) in a medium-sized bowl. In a separate medium-sized bowl, mix the liquid ingredients (coconut milk, canola oil, vinegar, and applesauce) together with the carrots. Add liquid ingredients to dry ingredients, and stir by hand until thoroughly combined. Allow to sit for 20 minutes covered.

Spray a glass pan (8 x 8-inch or 9 x 7-inch) with cooking spray, or spray 12 cup liners in a muffin baking pan. Remove all batter from the bowl with a spatula and spread uniformly in the pan or in equal amounts to each muffin cup. Bake at 400°F (204°C) for 20 minutes.

Servings: 12   **Serving size:** 1 corn muffin (60 grams)

Recommend with: Southern Black-eyed Peas or any meal.

Notes:
1. May substitute plant butter for canola oil. Heat butter in a microwave oven for 15 seconds to melt before adding to the plant milk.
2. May use unsweetened almond milk or unsweetened soymilk in place of coconut milk.

Nutrients Per Serving: 188 calories, 10 grams fat, 1 gram saturated fat, 2 grams protein, 21 grams carbohydrate, 1 grams fiber, 148 milligrams sodium

Parsley Mashed Potatoes

Parsley Mashed Potatoes go well with Spiced Beanloaf and many other dishes. For variations, try seasoning the potatoes with other herbs such as rosemary, thyme, oregano, chives, or sage.

3 pounds baking potatoes	(1,360 grams)
from about 7-8 potatoes, 2 by 4 inches each	
3 tablespoons plant butter	(40 grams)
1 cup (240 milliliters) unsweetened coconut milk	(230 grams)
refrigerated or boxed type, not canned, about 60 calories per cup	
or unsweetened almond milk	
1 teaspoon table salt	(6 grams)
½ teaspoon black pepper	(1 grams)
¼ cup finely chopped fresh Italian parsley	(15 grams)
Fresh Italian parsley leaves or twigs for garnish (optional)	

Wash and scrub potatoes thoroughly with water. Remove any bad spots (eyes or greenish areas on or just under the skin) on the potatoes. Otherwise, keep the skin intact. Cut potatoes into quarters by making one cross-sectional and one longitudinal cut. Add potatoes to a large stockpot with enough water to cover the potatoes. Bring to a boil and then turn down to a strong simmer for 30 minutes. Do not over boil or allow potatoes to remain in water for long after cooking is complete.

While the potatoes are simmering, place the butter in a microwave-safe glass container that holds at least 2 cups. Cover with a paper towel and heat in the microwave oven for about 30 seconds. Add the coconut milk and heat for another 30 seconds. Set aside.

Use a fork to test whether the potatoes are soft enough to mash. Remove from heat and drain off the water. Distribute the coconut milk, butter, salt, and pepper evenly over the potatoes. Scrape with a spatula to ensure transfer of all coconut milk and butter. Mash potatoes with a hand mixer to create a lumpy smooth texture. Stir in ¼ cup chopped parsley.

Replace the lid on the stockpot and keep covered to maintain warmth until potatoes are served. Garnish with a few parsley leaves or twigs when serving.

Servings: 7   **Serving size:** 1 cup (240 grams)

Recommend with: Spiced Beanloaf, Buttered Sweet Peas, or any meal.

Notes:
1. Chop parsley ahead of time and store in the refrigerator.
2. Select fresh potatoes with no green tints just under the skin. If green areas are found, be sure to remove those areas.

Nutrients Per Serving: 194 calories, 5 grams fat, 2 grams saturated fat, 4 grams protein, 34 grams carbohydrate, 3 grams fiber, 397 milligrams sodium

Sauteed Asparagus Spears

Sauteed asparagus is a quickly prepared side dish that accompanies many recipes well. I often serve it with falafels. A lemon wedge on each serving makes for a pretty garnish and offers a bit more zip to this dish.

32 very thin asparagus spears, trimmed to about 5 inches or 16 medium-thick spears	(95 grams)
1 teaspoon (5 milliliters) extra virgin olive oil	(5 grams)
1/16 teaspoon table salt	(<1 gram)
Lemon wedge (optional)	

Trim off the woody base ends of the asparagus to make a spear about 5 inches in length. Add olive oil to a 10-inch saute pan and heat to medium-high. Once oil is heated, add the asparagus spears. Use tongs to move the asparagus around in the pan to ensure even cooking. Sprinkle salt on spears while cooking. Saute until the asparagus is tender but not mushy. This takes about 3 minutes for very thin spears and about 5 minutes for medium-thick spears. Remove from heat. Serve with lemon wedge garnish.

Servings: 4   **Serving size:** 8 stalks (25 grams)

Recommend with: Spiced Beanloaf, Falafels with Tzatziki Sauce, or any meal.

Notes:
1. Do not overcook. Remove from heat when tender.

Nutrients Per Serving: 15 calories, 1 gram fat, 0 grams saturated fat, 1 gram protein, 1 gram carbohydrate, 0 grams fiber, 37 milligrams sodium

Seasonal Fresh Fruit Medley

The fruits in this recipe have been selected for their complementary flavors and widespread familiarity. This assortment may be freely modified to reflect seasonal availability, to add color to your table, or to include your own favorite fruit. For feeding large groups, add a seedless watermelon to the mix. Have one or two very large food grade plastic storage containers available to use for this recipe. Once the chopping is done, you will have a bountiful supply of ready-to-eat fruit for your future meals.

8 cups fresh cantaloupe chunks (1½-inch sides)	(1,190 grams)
from about 1 average size cantaloupe	
8 cups fresh honeydew melon chunks (1½-inch sides)	(1,110 grams)
from about 1 average size honeydew	
6 cups fresh pineapple chunks (1½-inch sides)	(760 grams)
from about 1 traditional pineapple	
4 cups destemmed red seedless grapes	(630 grams)
or cut small twigs instead of destemming	
3 cups halved (leaf tops removed) strawberries	(420 grams)
about 16 ounces	

Wash, drain and prepare all fruit. Place in a large storage container and refrigerate. Serve with meals or as a snack during the week.

Servings: 27   **Serving size:** 1 cup (150 grams)

Recommend with: any meal or snack.

Notes:
1. If apples are used, coat the slices with lemon juice to prevent browning.

Nutrients Per Serving: 65 calories, 0 grams fat, 0 grams saturated fat, 1 gram protein, 17 grams carbohydrate, 2 grams fiber, 15 milligrams sodium

Spring Side Salad

This is a great side salad that goes well with any dish. Use your favorite dressing or the one suggested here.

Dressing

2 tablespoons (30 milliliters) balsamic vinegar	(30 grams)
2 tablespoons (30 milliliters) extra virgin olive oil	(25 grams)

Salad

4 cups spring mix salad greens	(85 grams)
½ cup large-grated carrots	(55 grams)
½ cup julienne sliced yellow baby bell peppers	(55 grams)
2 tablespoons sliced in thin rounds and quartered radishes	(15 grams)
1 medium Hass avocado, sliced in strips or chunks	(135 grams)
4 teaspoons walnut pieces (optional)	(10 grams)

For the dressing: Whisk together the vinegar and oil. Set aside.

For the salad: Add 1 cup salad greens to each salad plate or bowl. Whisk the vinegar and oil again, and drizzle one tablespoon dressing over each plated salad greens. Add 2 tablespoons of carrots and 2 tablespoons of bell peppers to each plate. Sprinkle radishes onto the salad or place near the edge of each plate.

Prepare the avocado as close to serving time as possible to minimize discoloration. Using a paring knife, quarter the avocado by making four lengthwise slices through the rough skin down to the seed. Use the knife as a wedge between slices to release the pieces from the seed. Discard the seed, and peel and discard the outer avocado skin. Cut the avocado quarters into thinner slices or into chunks. Add ¼ of the avocado slices or chunks to each salad.

Add 1 teaspoon walnut pieces to each salad.

Servings: 4   **Serving size:** ¼ of salad (100 grams)

Recommend with: Red and White Pizzas, Savory Spaghetti, Chili de Verduras, or any meal.

Notes:
1. Add other garden vegetables, seeds, or nuts to make your own combination.

2. Watch a how-to video from the internet to observe how to cut an avocado or julienne vegetables.
3. Spring mix salad greens include several varieties of leafy greens and are widely available, premixed and prewashed, in salad packages.

Nutrients Per Serving: 153 calories, 14 grams fat, 2 grams saturated fat, 2 grams protein, 7 grams carbohydrate, 4 grams fiber, 24 milligrams sodium

Super Slaw

While Super Slaw is great as a side for many recipes, one of my favorites is with my Lentillies recipe. Pre-diced packages of cabbage (or cabbage and carrots) can be used to easily prepare this healthy, delicious side in just a few minutes.

1 pound (about 4 cups packed) diced cabbage pre-packaged diced or shredded cabbage works well	(440 grams)
½ cup plant mayonnaise	(110 grams)
1 tablespoon (15 milliliters) lemon juice	(15 grams)
1 tablespoon granulated sugar	(15 grams)
⅛ teaspoon table salt	(1 gram)
⅛ teaspoon black pepper	(<1 gram)

Utilizing pre-packaged diced or shredded cabbage saves time. Otherwise, dice cabbage at home using a food processor or by hand. Place cabbage in a bowl.

In a separate bowl, combine all other ingredients using a whisk or fork to combine. Then, stir the combination into the cabbage until well mixed. Refrigerate until ready to serve.

Servings: 8   **Serving size:** ½ cup (75 grams)

Recommend with: Lentilly sandwiches or any meal.

Nutrients Per Serving: 89 calories, 7 grams fat, 1 gram saturated fat, 1 gram protein, 7 grams carbohydrate, 1 gram fiber, 97 milligrams sodium

Tabouli Salad

This nutrient-dense Tabouli Salad features quinoa instead of cracked wheat. It is a perfect complement as a side to many dishes.

½ cup dried chickpeas or 15 ounces canned	(100 grams)
¼ cup plus 1 tablespoon dried quinoa, rinsed	(55 grams)
1 cup chopped (½-inch sides) fresh tomatoes	(180 grams)
1 cup packed finely chopped Italian parsley	(60 grams)
¼ cup packed finely chopped mint leaves	(6 grams)
¼ cup sliced (¼-inch thick rounds) scallions	(25 grams)
2 tablespoons (30 milliliters) extra virgin olive oil	(25 grams)
2 tablespoons (30 milliliters) lime juice	(30 grams)
⅛ teaspoon table salt	(1 gram)
⅛ teaspoon black pepper	(<1 gram)

Start dried chickpeas ahead of time using the overnight or quick soak method. After soaking, drain and discard water. Add plenty of fresh water, bring chickpeas to a boil and then turn down to a simmer for 1-1½ hours until chickpeas are tender. Remove from heat, drain, and cool.

Boil canned chickpeas with liquid from the can in a saucepan for 5 minutes. Remove from heat, drain and set aside to cool completely.

In a saucepan, add 1 cup water and quinoa. Bring to a boil. Cover with a lid and turn down to a simmer until water has been absorbed (usually about 15 minutes). Set aside to cool completely.

Add chickpeas, quinoa, tomatoes, parsley, mint, and scallions to a medium-sized bowl. In a separate bowl, mix together olive oil, lime juice, salt, and pepper. Sprinkle the oil mixture onto the other ingredients. Use a spatula to swipe the oil bowl clean. Stir the salad gently with a spoon. Refrigerate to chill.

Servings: 8   **Serving size:** ½ cup (90 grams)

Recommend with: Night on the Mediterranean Gyro or any meal.

Nutrients Per Serving: 114 calories, 5 grams fat, 1 gram saturated fat, 4 grams protein, 15 grams carbohydrate, 4 grams fiber, 45 milligrams sodium

Lunch Recipes

Broccoli, Apple, Walnut Salad   153
Butter Bean and Corn Salad   154
Chickpea Chia Salad   155
Crisp Vegetables and Hummus Sandwich   157
Lady Pea Salad   159
Quinoa Black Bean Bowl with Mango and Kale   160
Wild West Dip with Chips   162

Broccoli, Apple, Walnut Salad

This easy and refreshing salad makes a perfect lunch or side. Pack this salad for a healthy option in school lunch boxes or picnic baskets.

½ cup dried chickpeas or 15 ounces canned	(100 grams)
½ cup (120 milliliters) extra virgin olive oil	(110 grams)
¼ cup (60 milliliters) apple cider vinegar	(60 grams)
2 tablespoons granulated sugar	(25 grams)
½ teaspoon table salt	(3 grams)
3 cups chopped (¾-inch sides) apples	(375 grams)
6 cups cut (1-inch pieces) fresh broccoli florets	(550 grams)
½ cup walnut pieces	(60 grams)

Dried chickpeas require soaking. Place dried chickpeas in a stockpot, and cover the peas generously with water. Soak overnight or for at least 6-8 hours. Drain soaking water. Cover the peas with plenty of fresh water and bring to a boil. Turn down to a strong simmer for 1½-2 hours until chickpeas reach the desired tenderness (soft but not mushy/overcooked). Drain and set aside. When peas have cooled, place in a refrigerator.

For canned chickpeas: Add chickpeas and liquid from the can to a saucepan, and bring to a boil for 5 minutes. Remove from heat. Drain, cool, and refrigerate.

Mix olive oil, vinegar, sugar, and salt together in a bowl, and add the apples. Turn the apples to coat them. Combine the apples with the chickpeas and broccoli. Add walnuts. Serve chilled.

Servings: 10   **Serving size:** 1 cup (120 grams)

Recommend with: quinoa or whole-grain crackers, fresh fruit, and plant milk.

Notes:
1. Wash and cut broccoli in advance to save cooking time.
2. May use sliced almonds in place of walnuts. Toast almonds lightly at 350°F (177°C) for about 10 minutes.

Nutrients Per Serving: 224 calories, 16 grams fat, 2 grams saturated fat, 5 grams protein, 19 grams carbohydrate, 5 grams fiber, 139 milligrams sodium

Butter Bean and Corn Salad

This simple-to-make salad is a nutrient-dense, tasty, and colorful stand-alone meal. Double the recipe ingredients for larger groups or to make additional servings for use later in the week. My favorite variety of corn for this recipe is Shoepeg.

2 cups frozen butter beans or baby lima beans	(330 grams)
2 cups frozen cut white corn kernels	(330 grams)
⅓ cup plant mayonnaise	(75 grams)
½ teaspoon table salt	(3 grams)
½ teaspoon black pepper	(1 gram)
4 cups spring mix salad greens	(85 grams)
2 cups grape tomatoes	(300 grams)

Place the butter or lima beans in a stockpot, and immerse the beans in water. Bring to a boil and turn down to a simmer (covered) for 30 minutes. Add the corn to the beans. Heat on high for 2 minutes. Remove from heat and drain. Place beans and corn in a bowl. Add mayonnaise, salt, and pepper. Mix by hand to distribute ingredients evenly. Allow to cool, and place in the refrigerator until time to serve.

For each serving, create a bed of 1 cup spring mix greens or lettuce. Place one cup of bean and corn mixture on the greens/lettuce bed. Top with ½ cup grape tomatoes or as much as you like.

Servings: 4   **Serving size:** 1 cup greens or lettuce, 1 cup bean and corn mixture, ½ cup tomatoes (210 grams)

Recommend with: whole-grain crackers, fresh fruit, and plant milk.

Nutrients Per Serving: 289 calories, 10 grams fat, 2 grams saturated fat, 10 grams protein, 44 grams carbohydrate, 8 grams fiber, 418 milligrams sodium

Chickpea Chia Salad

Enjoy this crisp, and refreshingly chilled chickpea salad any time of the year. Use this protein and fiber rich recipe as either a main or a side dish.

1 cup dried chickpeas (garbanzo beans) or 30 ounces canned	(200 grams)
2 cups peeled and diced (¼-inch sides) celery lightly peel fibrous outer layer	(260 grams)
1 teaspoon plant chicken flavor bouillon base or cube for 1 cup equivalent, do not reconstitute	(6 grams)
5 tablespoons (75 milliliters) lemon juice, divided	(75 grams)
½ cup plant mayonnaise	(110 grams)
1 tablespoon black chia seeds	(10 grams)
⅛ teaspoon table salt	(1 gram)
¼ teaspoon black pepper	(1 gram)

Topping
Walnut halves and pieces (optional)

Use the overnight soaking method to prepare dried chickpeas. After soaking, drain and then cover the chickpeas with plenty of fresh water. Bring to a boil and then turn down to a strong simmer for 1-1½ hours until peas become tender. Drain and set aside. Refrigerate chickpeas that you are not using right away.

Boil canned chickpeas with the liquid from the can in a saucepan for 5 minutes. Remove from heat, drain and set aside to cool.

Remove the tough outer coating from the celery stalk using a vegetable peeler and dice the stalk. Set aside.

Add bouillon base to 1 tablespoon of lemon juice. If a bouillon cube is used, as needed, heat the bouillon and lemon juice in a microwave oven for 10 seconds to help dissolve the bouillon. Combine the remaining lemon juice, mayonnaise, chia seeds, salt, and pepper in a mixing bowl with the bouillon. Stir in the chickpeas and diced celery. Refrigerate for at least 2 hours. Serve chilled.

For the topping: Top each serving with a few walnut pieces if desired.

Servings: 4   **Serving size:** 1 cup (200 grams)

Recommend with: mixed salad greens, whole-grain crackers, fresh fruit, and plant milk.

Notes:
1. Peel and dice celery ahead of time and store in the refrigerator.
2. Make the recipe ahead of time and refrigerate for lunches or sides for the next few days ahead.
3. For non-plant-based eaters add a baked chicken breast or tenderloin torn into very small pieces for individual servings.

Nutrients Per Serving: 318 calories, 15 grams fat, 2 grams saturated fat, 10 grams protein, 37 grams carbohydrate, 10 grams fiber, 339 milligrams sodium

Crisp Vegetables and Hummus Sandwich

Enjoy this fresh and tasty sandwich that can be made with either a ciabatta or hoagie-style bread roll. Use whole-grain bread when available. The combination of vegetables with seasoned rice vinegar gives this sandwich a delightful, piquant flavor.

¼ cup sliced black olives in ¼-inch thick rounds	(35 grams)
¼ cup sliced, mild, pickled banana peppers	(40 grams)
½ cup julienne sliced sweet mini peppers	(55 grams)
¼ cup julienne sliced purple onions	(30 grams)
1 cup spring mix salad greens or lettuce leaves	(20 grams)
8 tomato slices	(150 grams)
from about 2 medium tomatoes	
8 cucumber slices in ¼-inch thick rounds	(40 grams)
4 whole-grain ciabatta bread rolls	(200 grams)
or 6-inch whole-grain hoagie rolls	
4 ounces sliced plant provolone cheese	(90 grams)
½ cup prepared hummus	(120 grams)
or make your own (Classic Hummus recipe under "Sides")	
¼ cup (60 milliliters) seasoned or sweet rice wine vinegar	(55 grams)
⅛ teaspoon table salt	(1 gram)
⅛ teaspoon ground black pepper	(<1 gram)

Wash and prepare vegetables (olives, banana peppers, sweet mini peppers, onions, salad greens, tomatoes, and cucumbers) and place separately on a plate.

Prepare ciabatta or hoagie rolls for sandwiches by using a bread knife to slice the rolls horizontally into top and bottom halves. Place both halves on an oven pan with the cut surfaces facing upward. Place cheese slices on the top half of each roll. Lightly toast both halves of each roll (top half with cheese, bottom half without).

To assemble, spread 2 tablespoons of hummus on the half of each roll that is not covered by cheese. Place vegetables on top of the hummus to help the vegetables stay in place. In the following order, add 1 tablespoon olives, 1 tablespoon banana peppers, 2 tablespoons pepper strips, 1 tablespoon onions, ¼ cup spring mix or lettuce leaves, 2 tomato slices, and 2 cucumber slices to each sandwich. Sprinkle 1 tablespoon seasoned or sweet rice vinegar over the vegetables on each sandwich. Sprinkle salt and pepper over open sandwiches. Place the top (cheese) half of the roll on the bottom (vegetable) half to close the sandwiches. Enjoy!

Servings: 4   **Serving size:** 1 sandwich (210 grams)

Recommend with: whole-grain pita bread wedges with extra hummus, fresh fruit, and plant milk.

Notes:
1. Prepare vegetables ahead of time.

Nutrients Per Serving: 309 calories, 12 grams fat, 5 grams saturated fat, 5 grams protein, 46 grams carbohydrate, 8 grams fiber, 830 milligrams sodium

Lady Pea Salad

This lady pea recipe is best served chilled. It is fresh and delicious when served over a small bed of spring salad greens with a few whole-grain crackers. This recipe makes enough for leftovers to enjoy on another day. It is also a perfect dish to serve on a picnic! Use frozen or dried lady peas, lady cream peas, zipper peas, or butter peas.

4 cups cooked lady peas	(720 grams)
⅓ cup plant mayonnaise	(75 grams)
1 tablespoon nutritional yeast	(5 grams)
½ teaspoon prepared yellow mustard	(3 grams)
½ teaspoon table salt	(3 grams)
½ teaspoon black pepper	(1 grams)
½ teaspoon turmeric	(1 grams)
¼ cup sliced (¼-inch thick rounds) scallions	(25 grams)
2 tablespoons (30 milliliters) lemon juice	(60 grams)

Cook fresh, frozen, or dried lady peas according to package directions. Do not overcook. Drain and set aside. Refrigerate when peas have cooled.

Combine the mayonnaise, yeast, mustard, salt, pepper, and turmeric together. Add the scallions and lemon juice.

Mix peas with the other ingredients. Refrigerate until ready to serve.

Servings: 4   **Serving size:** 1 cup (220 grams)

Recommend with: spring mix salad greens, pickle spear, whole-grain crackers, fresh fruit, and plant milk.

Notes:
1. If using dried lady cream peas: 1½ cups dried lady cream peas yields approximately 4 cups cooked.

Nutrients Per Serving: 301 calories, 10 grams fat, 2 grams saturated fat, 14 grams protein, 41 grams carbohydrate, 12 grams fiber, 379 milligrams sodium

Quinoa Black Bean Bowl with Mango and Kale

This delicious and refreshingly chilled recipe can be served as a main dish or as a side. One of the main ingredients in this recipe is quinoa which is gluten-free. Leftovers can be stored in the refrigerator for about 4 days.

1 cup plus 4 teaspoons dried black beans	(210 grams)
1 cup dried quinoa, rinsed in a fine-mesh strainer	(170 grams)
3 cups peeled and chopped (½-inch sides) mango from about 2 large mangos	(450 grams)
5 ounces fresh baby kale, finely chopped from about 10 cups unchopped	(140 grams)
⅓ cup (80 milliliters) unfiltered apple cider vinegar	(80 grams)
3 tablespoons (45 milliliters) extra virgin olive oil	(40 grams)
2 tablespoons (30 milliliters) lime juice	(30 grams)
1½ teaspoon granulated sugar	(6 grams)
½ teaspoon table salt	(3 grams)

Soak dried black beans overnight or for 6-8 hours in a stockpot with a generous covering of water. Drain soaking water. Cover with plenty of fresh water and bring to a boil. Turn down to a strong simmer for 45 minutes to 1 hour until the beans are tender. Drain and set aside. Allow beans to cool, then place in the refrigerator.

Add 2 cups of water to a saucepan and bring to a boil. Add quinoa to boiling water. Cover with lid and turn down to a simmer. Simmer for 15-20 minutes. Remove from heat and set aside. When cooled, place in the refrigerator.

Place chopped mango and baby kale in separate containers in the refrigerator to chill.

In a large bowl, add the chilled black beans, quinoa, mango, and kale. Separately, mix vinegar, olive oil, lime juice, sugar, and salt together. Pour the vinegar and oil mixture over the quinoa and beans mixture, and stir until evenly distributed.

Servings: 10   **Serving size:** 1 cup (180 grams)

Recommend with: fresh fruit and plant milk.

Notes:
1. To save time, cut mango ahead of cooking time and store it in the refrigerator. May cook quinoa and beans ahead of time and store them in the refrigerator as well.
2. Try topping with a sprinkle of toasted almonds.

Nutrients Per Serving: 202 calories, 5 grams fat, 1 gram saturated fat, 8 grams protein, 32 grams carbohydrate, 7 grams fiber, 123 milligrams sodium

Wild West Dip with Chips

This mighty dip is great with tortilla chips, tacos, or enchiladas. Be careful not to overcook the peas, beans, and corn.

½ cup dried black-eyed peas or 15 ounces canned	(90 grams)
½ cup plus 2 teaspoons dried black beans or 15 ounces canned	(100 grams)
1½ cups frozen cut white corn kernels	(240 grams)
2½ cups quartered grape tomatoes	(450 grams)
½ cup diced (¼-inch sides) green bell peppers	(75 grams)
⅓ cup diced (¼-inch sides) purple onions	(55 grams)
¼ cup finely chopped cilantro leaves	(4 grams)
1 tablespoon deseeded, minced jalapeno peppers	(6 grams)
⅓ cup (80 milliliters) extra virgin olive oil	(70 grams)
3 tablespoons (45 milliliters) lime juice	(45 grams)
1 tablespoon plus 2 teaspoons (25 milliliters) apple cider vinegar	(25 grams)
1 tablespoon granulated sugar	(15 grams)
½ teaspoon table salt	(3 grams)
7 ounces tortilla chips, about 15 chips per serving	(230 grams)

Use the overnight soaking method to prepare the dried black-eyed peas and dried black beans. Soak the peas and beans separately since black beans may discolor black-eyed peas. Drain. In separate pots cover the peas and beans with plenty of fresh water. Bring each to a boil and then turn down to a strong simmer for about 45 minutes to 1 hour until peas and beans are tender. Watch progress to assure that peas and beans are not undercooked (too firm) or overcooked (too soft/mushy). Drain and set aside. When cool, refrigerate any peas or beans that you are not using right away.

For canned black-eyed peas, place the peas with the liquid from the can in a pot and bring to a boil. Turn heat down to a simmer and continue for 5 minutes. Remove from heat. Drain and allow to cool. Repeat the same process for canned black beans. Heat the peas and beans in separate pots to prevent the black beans from discoloring the black-eyed peas.

Place corn in a saucepan and add about 1 cup of water. Bring to a boil for 2-3 minutes. Drain and allow to cool.

After the peas, beans, and corn have cooled completely, add the peas, beans, corn, tomatoes, bell peppers, onions, cilantro, and jalapeno to a bowl. In a separate bowl, whisk together the olive oil, lime juice, vinegar, sugar, and salt until the solids have dissolved. Add the liquid to the peas and beans mixture, and gently fold to combine. Chill in the refrigerator until time to serve.

Servings: 7   **Serving size:** 1 cup (190 grams), 1 ounce tortilla chips (30 grams)

Recommend with: tortilla chips, lettuce greens, fresh fruit, and plant milk.

Notes:
1. To save time, cook and refrigerate peas and beans in advance.
2. May use canned corn in place of frozen corn.

Nutrients Per Serving: 358 calories, 17 grams fat, 2 grams saturated fat, 10 grams protein, 45 grams carbohydrate, 9 grams fiber, 168 milligrams sodium

Breakfast Recipes

Bagels with Seed Butter and Berries   165
Banana Muffins   166
Blueberry Muffins   168
Good-Morning Grits   170
Heavenly Hash Browns and Black Beans   172
Overnight Oats with Peaches   174
Perfect Pancakes or Waffles   175

Bagels with Seed Butter and Berries

This recipe offers many options and is not only delicious but also quick, easy, and loaded with nutrients—exactly what you need in the morning. Choose your favorite berry or berry combination. You can't go wrong!

2 cups fresh single or assorted berries	(290 grams)
4 whole-grain bagels	(390 grams)
about 3.5 ounces (100 grams) each	
½ cup sunflower (or other) seed butter	(130 grams)
4 tablespoons sliced almonds	(25 grams)
1 teaspoon brown sugar (optional)	(5 grams)

Servings: 4   **Serving size:** 1 bagel with toppings (210 grams)

Rinse and drain berries, and set aside. Open bagels and lightly oven toast the open faces. Scoop your favorite seed butter into a bowl and add brown sugar if desired. Spread 2 tablespoons seed butter (and brown sugar) on toasted faces of each bagel. Sprinkle 1 tablespoon almonds over the seed butter. Top with berries.

Recommend with: plant milk or orange juice fortified with calcium.

Notes:
1. May also substitute your favorite nut butter in place of seed butter, and walnuts or other nuts in place of almonds.
2. If berries are not readily available try topping with chopped prunes. Delicious!

Nutrients Per Serving: 513 calories, 22 grams fat, 2 grams saturated fat, 17 grams protein, 66 grams carbohydrate, 9 grams fiber, 432 milligrams sodium

Banana Muffins

These muffins are both delicious and versatile. The recipe makes 24 small or 12 large muffins that can easily be frozen and reheated. To reheat, microwave two frozen muffins for 20 seconds and then heat in an oven or toaster oven on 200 °F (95 °C) until the muffins are warmed throughout.

2 cups (470 milliliters) mashed bananas from about 5 medium or 4 large bananas	(450 grams)
1 cup rolled oats	(160 grams)
2 tablespoons ground flaxseed	(15 grams)
½ cup (120 milliliters) canola oil	(110 grams)
⅓ cup (80 milliliters) water	(80 grams)
1 tablespoon (15 milliliters) lemon juice	(15 grams)
2 cups all-purpose flour	(250 grams)
¾ cup granulated sugar	(150 grams)
1 tablespoon baking powder	(15 grams)
½ teaspoon baking soda	(3 grams)
½ teaspoon salt	(3 grams)
Cooking spray	
1 tablespoon coarse sugar, divided ¼ teaspoon for each large or ⅛ teaspoon for each small muffin	(25 grams)
⅓ cup chopped walnut pieces, divided (optional) from 6 whole walnuts, divided into 12 walnut halves for large or 24 walnut fourths for small muffins	(40 grams)

Peel bananas and mash in a large bowl. Stir in the oats and ground flaxseed. Add canola oil, water, and lemon juice to the banana and oats mixture. Stir until combined. Allow the ingredients to rest for 10 minutes. This rest is important to help the mixture reach the correct consistency. In a separate mixing bowl, combine the flour, sugar, baking powder, baking soda, and salt. Add this to the banana and oat mixture. Place paper liners in the cups of a muffin pan, and spray the liner interiors with cooking spray. Pour batter evenly into each muffin cup. Sprinkle coarse sugar and walnuts on top of each muffin. Bake at 350°F (177°C) for 20-25 minutes for small muffins and 30-35 minutes for large muffins. Rotate the pan 180 degrees midway through baking.

Servings: 12   **Serving size:** 2 small or 1 large muffin (100 grams)

Recommend with: fresh fruit, and plant milk or orange juice fortified with calcium.

Notes:
1. Mix dry ingredients together ahead of time.
2. Use standard or regular-sized paper liners for small muffins and large liners for large muffins.

Nutrients Per Serving: 321 calories, 13 grams fat, 1 gram saturated fat, 6 grams protein, 48 grams carbohydrate, 3 grams fiber, 243 milligrams sodium

Blueberry Muffins

Fresh blueberries turn this recipe into an all-time family favorite. The muffins can be easily frozen and reheated. To reheat, microwave two frozen muffins for 20 seconds and then heat them in an oven or toaster oven on 200 °F (95 °C) until the muffins are warmed throughout.

1 cup rolled oats	(160 grams)
2 tablespoons ground flaxseed	(15 grams)
1 cup (240 milliliters) unsweetened coconut milk	(230 grams)
refrigerated or boxed type, not canned, about 60 calories per cup	
½ cup (120 milliliters) canola oil	(110 grams)
1 tablespoon (15 milliliters) lemon juice	(15 grams)
2 cups all-purpose flour	(250 grams)
¾ cup granulated sugar	(150 grams)
1 tablespoon baking powder	(15 grams)
½ teaspoon baking soda	(3 grams)
½ teaspoon salt	(3 grams)
2 cups fresh blueberries	(290 grams)
Cooking spray	
2 tablespoons coarse sugar, divided	(25 grams)
½ teaspoon for each large or ¼ teaspoon for each small muffin	
⅓ cup almond slices, divided (optional)	(30 grams)

Mix the oats and flaxseed together in a large bowl. Add the coconut milk, canola oil, and lemon juice to the oats and flaxseed, and stir until combined. Allow the ingredients to rest for 10 minutes to permit the mixture to reach the correct consistency. In a separate mixing bowl, combine the flour, sugar, baking powder, baking soda, and salt. Add this to the oat, flaxseed, and milk ingredients. Wash the blueberries and drain well. Fold the blueberries into the existing mix. Place paper liners in the cups of a muffin pan, and spray the liner interiors with cooking spray. Pour batter evenly into each muffin cup. Sprinkle coarse sugar and almond slices on each muffin top. Bake at 350°F (177°C) for 20-25 minutes for small muffins and 30-35 minutes for large muffins. Rotate the pan 180 degrees midway through baking.

Servings: 12   **Serving size:** 2 small or 1 large muffin (100 grams)

Recommend with: fresh fruit, and plant milk or orange juice fortified with calcium.

Notes:
1. Mix dry ingredients together in advance to reduce cooking time.
2. Use muffin cups with cooking spray to prevent the muffins from falling apart when removed from the muffin pan.
3. Use standard or regular-sized paper liners for small muffins and large liners for large muffins.

Nutrients Per Serving: 305 calories, 12 grams fat, 1 gram saturated fat, 5 grams protein, 44 grams carbohydrate, 3 grams fiber, 247 milligrams sodium

Good-Morning Grits

Grits are great in the morning, and there are many ways to enjoy grits at any time of the day. This recipe is very simple and can easily be used at any meal. Try adding side items such as tomato slices, plant sausage, a spring salad with poppy seed dressing, or steamed broccoli that reflect the time of day. Mix in plant cheeses to make cheese grits.

1 cup cut fresh cauliflower florets in ½-inch pieces	(105 grams)
2 cups (470 milliliters) water	(470 grams)
2 cups (470 milliliters) almond milk	(480 grams)
¼ cup plant butter	(55 grams)
¼ teaspoon table salt	(2 grams)
¼ teaspoon black pepper	(1 gram)
1 cup 5-minute quick grits	(160 grams)

Place cauliflower into a saucepan and cover the cauliflower with water. Bring to a boil and turn down to a simmer with lid in place for 10 minutes. Drain with a strainer. Return the cauliflower to the saucepan. Mash cauliflower to a smooth consistency with a potato masher.

Add 2 cups water, almond milk, butter, salt, and pepper to the saucepan containing cauliflower. Bring to a simmer and sprinkle grits evenly into the pan to avoid lump formations. Continue to simmer (covered) for 5 minutes, stirring every minute to ensure the grits are not sticking to the bottom of the pan. Keep pan covered with lid when not stirring. Remove from heat and serve while hot.

Servings: 5   **Serving size:** 1 cup (240 grams)

Recommend with: tomato slices, fresh fruit, and orange juice fortified with calcium.

Notes:
1. If there are leftovers, try pouring the grits into a tall, smooth, cylindrical drinking glass, and refrigerate. On the next day, turn the glass over, and the grits will slide out in the shape of a perfect cylinder. Slice into ½-inch thick rounds. Heat a fry pan on medium heat and spray with cooking spray. Heat the grits cakes several minutes on each side until golden, turning only once to avoid having grits stick to the pan.
2. To please non-plant-based eaters, consider adding cheddar cheese to grits.

Nutrients Per Serving: 201 calories, 9 grams fat, 2 grams saturated fat, 3 grams protein, 27 grams carbohydrate, 2 grams fiber, 271 milligrams sodium

Heavenly Hash Browns and Black Beans

This easy recipe may be enjoyed at any meal and is sure to please. Follow these two steps during cooking to ensure a good result. First, heat the pan to cooking temperature before adding the hash browns. And second, check the hash browns closely until you see that they are browned on one side and then turn them only one time.

Black beans

½ cup plus 2 teaspoons dried black beans or 15 ounces canned	(100 grams)
½ cup (120 milliliters) water (dried beans only) for canned beans, use liquid from the can instead	(120 grams)
¼ cup chopped (½-inch sides) yellow or sweet onions	(40 grams)

Toppings

Cooking spray	
1 cup chopped (½-inch sides) yellow or sweet onions	(160 grams)
1 cup prepared salsa	(260 grams)
½ cup plant cheddar cheese	(55 grams)
½ cup plant sour cream	(110 grams)

Hash browns

¼ cup (60 milliliters) canola oil, divided	(55 grams)
8 cups (1 pound 7 ounces) frozen shredded hash browns cooks down to 4 cups	(660 grams)
⅛ teaspoon black pepper	(<1 gram)

For the beans: For dried black beans, use the overnight soaking method. Drain soaking water. Cover the beans with plenty of fresh water and bring to a boil. Turn down to a strong simmer for 45 minutes to 1 hour until beans are tender. Drain and set aside. When cooled, place in the refrigerator.

Canned beans are used directly from the can without soaking or preliminary cooking.

Add beans, ½ cup water (or liquid from can), and ¼ cup onions to a saucepan. Simmer for 10 minutes just before serving. Add salt (optional) to taste.

For the toppings: Spray a saute pan with cooking spray and saute 1 cup onions until translucent and starting to brown. Remove from heat. Place all toppings (onions, salsa, cheddar cheese, and sour cream) in separate serving containers.

For the hash browns: Add 2 tablespoons canola oil to a large saute or frying pan. Heat oil to medium-high. Spread 4 cups frozen hash browns evenly in pan. Do not move the hash browns around once placed in the pan. Peek underneath frequently to check for desired browning and when reached, turn the hash browns one time. Sprinkle with black pepper. Add the toppings after the hash browns have been turned or when served.

Repeat the process using a second large saute or frying pan, or after scraping clean and drying the first pan.

Serve the hash browns and black beans separately on the same plate.

Servings: 4   **Serving size:** 1 cup hash browns (130 grams), ¼ of toppings (140 grams), ⅓ cup beans (100 grams)

Recommend with: sliced tomatoes or mixed salad greens, fresh fruit, and orange juice fortified with calcium.

Notes:
1. Add salt and pepper to taste.
2. Consider adding diced jalapeno peppers to hash browns for a spicy twist.
3. Save time by cutting onions in advance.

Nutrients Per Serving: 499 calories, 23 grams fat, 5 grams saturated fat, 12 grams protein, 66 grams carbohydrate, 10 grams fiber, 766 milligrams sodium

Overnight Oats with Peaches

Start these overnight oats before bedtime, and, in a snap, have them ready to serve for breakfast the next morning. They are good cold or hot. Using fresh fruit in this recipe is amazing, but frozen is a nice and convenient choice too. This recipe is nutrient dense with 6 grams of fiber and 8 grams of protein that will give you a great start on your day!

½ cup regular rolled oats, not quick 1-minute oats	(25 grams)
Pinch of salt (about 1/16 teaspoon)	(<1 gram)
½ cup (120 milliliters) unsweetened almond milk	(120 grams)
2 teaspoons maple syrup	(40 grams)
1 cup chopped (¾-inch pieces) peaches	(150 grams)
2 tablespoons chopped walnuts	(15 grams)

Recipe makes 1 serving. Double, triple, or quadruple ingredients to make 2-4 servings.

Start preparation on the night before breakfast. Combine oats and salt in a bowl. Add plant milk and syrup to the oats, and stir. Add frozen peaches or wait to add fresh peaches in the morning. Fold in walnuts at night or the morning. Refrigerate overnight in a covered container. Serve (cold) right from the refrigerator or serve (warm) by heating in a microwave oven for about 1½ minutes.

Servings: 1   **Serving size:** 1½ cups (350 grams)

Recommend with: plant milk or orange juice fortified with calcium.

Notes:
1. While peaches are called for in this recipe, have fun experimenting with apples, bananas, blueberries, or strawberries instead.
2. Sliced almonds may be used in place of walnuts.
3. Add ⅛ teaspoon of cinnamon for an additional breakfast flavor.

Nutrients Per Serving: 307 calories, 13 grams fat, 1 gram saturated fat, 8 grams protein, 43 grams carbohydrate, 6 grams fiber, 242 milligrams sodium

Perfect Pancakes (or Waffles)

What a great way to start your day! The sky's the limit with this versatile recipe. It was originally given to me by my dear Aunt Betty, and I have modified it to be plant-based. Select the toppings that you like best. Fresh berries and pecans are two of my favorite toppings, but others you might try include bananas, apples and cinnamon, cherry preserves, walnuts, almonds, or plant chocolate chips. If you have a waffle iron, reducing the plant milk to 1½ cups, turns this recipe for pancakes into a recipe for waffles!

Toppings selection

2 cups fresh berries	(290 grams)
(blackberries, blueberries, raspberries, or strawberries)	
½ cup pecan halves	(50 grams)
¼ cup powdered sugar	(30 grams)
or maple syrup	

Pancake mix

1½ cups all-purpose flour	(190 grams)
2½ teaspoons baking powder	(10 grams)
1 tablespoon flaxseed flour	(7 grams)
1 teaspoon granulated sugar	(4 grams)
½ teaspoon table salt	(3 grams)
1¾ cups (410 milliliters) unsweetened almond milk	(420 grams)
2 tablespoons (30 milliliters) canola oil	(25 grams)
2 teaspoons (10 milliliters) white vinegar	(10 grams)
Cooking spray	

For the toppings: Select and gather toppings in separate serving containers.

For the pancake mix: Mix dry pancake ingredients together in a bowl. In a separate bowl, add liquid ingredients. Combine liquid ingredients with dry ingredients. Use a whisk or fork to stir until lumpy smooth.

Heat a large skillet to medium heat. Add cooking spray. When the pan is heated (a hot pan is especially important if using stainless steel cookware), add ¼ cup of batter to the pan, for each of three pancakes. Heat for several minutes. When bubbles start to form on top of the pancake, check the underside by peeking with a thin spatula. When the underside is light golden, carefully flip the pancakes to the other side. Using a spatula, remove pancakes from the pan when both sides are golden and place on an individual or serving plate. Repeat the process until all batter has been cooked. Turn down heat to medium-low if the pan gets too hot after cooking several rounds of pancakes.

Spoon berries and/or pecan halves and/or pour maple syrup on individual servings. Dust powdered sugar over the pancakes through a small wire mesh strainer just before serving.

Servings: 4 **Serving size:** three, 4-inch pancakes with toppings (260 grams)

Recommend with: plant milk or orange juice fortified with calcium.

Notes:
1. Mix dry ingredients together and store in a sealed container to save time in the mornings.
2. Double the recipe for more pancakes.
3. Freeze leftover pancakes in three-pancake servings separated with parchment paper to pull out and heat in the microwave oven for a quick breakfast.
4. Add a little more plant milk if thinner pancakes are desired.

Nutrients Per Serving: 412 calories, 18 grams fat, 1 gram saturated fat, 8 grams protein, 56 grams carbohydrate, 6 grams fiber, 603 milligrams sodium

Beverage Recipes

Strawberry Dream Smoothie   178
Sunshine Smoothie   179

Strawberry Dream Smoothie

Reduce inflammation and support the health of your heart and skin with this dream smoothie rich in antioxidants, vitamins (including vitamin C) and minerals (including potassium). Feel rejuvenated in no time after having one of these!

1½ cups (360 milliliters) unsweetened soymilk	(360 grams)
1 cup baby spinach, rinsed and drained	(30 grams)
2 cups frozen strawberries	(300 grams)
1 cup frozen dark sweet cherries	(160 grams)
1 cup frozen pineapple chunks	(160 grams)

Add all ingredients into a blender. Blend until smooth.

Servings: 4 **Serving size:** 1 cup (240 grams)

Recommend with: any meal or snack.

Notes:
1. Use a different plant milk as desired.
2. If your blender does not handle frozen fruits well, allow the fruit to thaw a bit before blending.

Nutrients Per Serving: 100 calories, 2 grams fat, 0 grams saturated fat, 4 grams protein, 19 grams carbohydrate, 3 grams fiber, 41 milligrams sodium

Sunshine Smoothie

This refreshing smoothie will flood your body with antioxidants and phytonutrients, such as beta carotene and lutein, to support the health of your eyes, skin, and immune system. Each of the ingredients is essential to the perfect taste! This pick-me-up smoothie goes well with any meal or snack.

1 cup (240 milliliters) unsweetened soymilk	(240 grams)
½ cup (120 milliliters) orange juice	(120 grams)
1 cup baby carrots	(120 grams)
1 seedless mandarin orange, peeled	(75 grams)
1 cup frozen mango chunks	(170 grams)
1 cup frozen pineapple chunks	(160 grams)
2 ice cubes	(30 grams)

Add all ingredients into a blender. Blend until smooth. Place in the freezer for 10-15 minutes for a more frosted drink.

Servings: 4   **Serving size:** 1 cup (230 grams)

Recommend with: any meal or snack.

Notes:
1. Use a different plant milk if preferred.

Nutrients Per Serving: 100 calories, 1 gram fat, 0 grams saturated fat, 3 grams protein, 21 grams carbohydrate, 2 grams fiber, 47 milligrams sodium

Dessert Recipes

Apple Crisp   181
Chocolate Chip Oatmeal Cookies   183

Apple Crisp

This recipe reminds me of early Fall, although it can be enjoyed at any time of the year. Whether it is served for dessert or for breakfast, Apple Crisp is sure to be a favorite!

Oatmeal crisp
¾ cup packed dark brown sugar	(170 grams)
¾ cup all-purpose flour	(95 grams)
¾ cup regular rolled oats, not quick 1-minute oats	(40 grams)
½ teaspoon baking powder	(2 grams)
½ cup plant butter	(110 grams)
Cooking spray	

Apples
8 cups peeled Granny Smith apple chunks (¾-inch sides) from about 6-8 large apples	(880 grams)
½ teaspoon (3 milliliters) lemon juice	(3 grams)
1 tablespoon plant butter	(15 grams)
¼ cup packed dark brown sugar	(55 grams)
1 teaspoon cinnamon	(2 grams)
½ teaspoon cornstarch	(1 gram)

Toppings
½ cup walnut pieces — one walnut or 1 tablespoon of pieces per serving	(60 grams)
2 teaspoons coarse sugar — ¼ teaspoon per serving	(8 grams)

For the oatmeal crisp: Mix all dry ingredients (sugar, flour, oats, and baking powder) together in a mixing bowl. Add butter in small pieces evenly spread around the bowl. Using the back of a large spoon or your fingers (fingers work best), work the butter into the dry mix until saturated. Spray a 9 x 13-inch glass baking dish with cooking spray. Crumble and evenly spread the oatmeal mix in the baking dish. Bake at 350°F (177°C) for 12 minutes. Remove from the oven and allow the crisp to cool a bit. Using a large knife, divide the crisp into 8 rectangular squares.

For the apples: Add the apples, lemon juice, and butter to a large stockpot. Mix brown sugar, cinnamon, and cornstarch together in a bowl, and sprinkle the apples with the mix. Cover with a lid and heat the stockpot to medium heat. Continue to heat on medium for about 10-12 minutes.

Stir frequently and cover with lid when not stirring. If apples get too hot, turn heat to medium-low or low. When finished cooking, remove from heat and set aside. Apples should be tender but not mushy. Do not over or undercook.

Place ¾ cup of cooked apple mixture into a bowl. Sprinkle each serving of apples with ¼ teaspoon coarse sugar and one tablespoon walnut pieces. Place one oatmeal crisp rectangle on top.

Servings: 8 **Serving size:** ¾ cup apples, 1 oatmeal crisp (180 grams)

Recommend with: plant milk, coffee, or tea.

Notes:
1. Make the oatmeal crisp ahead of time and refrigerate until ready to cook.
2. When measuring brown sugar, use the back of a spoon to compact the sugar.

Nutrients Per Serving: 363 calories, 16 grams fat, 3 grams saturated fat, 3 grams protein, 56 grams carbohydrate, 3 grams fiber, 133 milligrams sodium

Chocolate Chip Oatmeal Cookies

Make sweet memories with this recipe. My favorite way to store chocolate chip cookies is to freeze them several hours after making them. That will keep them fresh for a long time. When you are ready for a treat, pull one out and allow it to sit at room temperature for 10 minutes or heat it in the microwave oven for 10 seconds. Yum!!

2 tablespoons ground flaxseed	(15 grams)
2 tablespoons (30 milliliters) water	(30 grams)
1½ cups all-purpose flour	(190 grams)
1 teaspoon baking soda	(5 grams)
1 teaspoon table salt	(6 grams)
1 cup packed dark brown sugar	(220 grams)
½ cup granulated sugar	(100 grams)
1 cup plant butter	(220 grams)
1 teaspoon (5 milliliters) vanilla extract	(4 grams)
2 cups regular rolled oats, **not quick 1-minute oats**	(310 grams)
10 ounces semi-sweet plant chocolate chips	(280 grams)
use mini size chips if available	
Cooking spray	

In a small bowl, stir together flaxseed and water, and set aside.

In a medium-sized bowl, combine all-purpose flour, baking soda, and salt, then set aside.

In a large bowl, stir the brown and white sugars together. Add butter, vanilla, and the flaxseed water mix (small bowl) to the sugar bowl, and beat these ingredients together using a hand mixer. Then, gradually beat in the all-purpose flour mixture (medium bowl) and the rolled oats. Stir in the chocolate chips by hand. Measure out 2 teaspoons of dough per cookie and space them 1-inch apart on a baking sheet sprayed with cooking spray or covered with parchment paper.

Bake at **350°F (177°C)** for 10-12 minutes. Remove cookies from the baking sheet and place on a wire rack to cool.

Servings: 36 (makes 108 cookies)   **Serving size:** 3 cookies (35 grams)

Recommend with: plant milk, coffee, or tea.

Notes:
1. Store cookies in the freezer to keep fresh and pull out the needed servings when you are ready to eat.

Nutrients Per Serving: 158 calories, 6 grams fat, 2 grams saturated fat, 2 grams protein, 23 grams carbohydrate, 1 gram fiber, 150 milligrams sodium

Appendix A
One Week of Sample Meals with the Weekly Menu Planner

One Week of Sample Meals

	Breakfast	Lunch	Supper
Sunday	Whole-grain Dry Cereal & Plant Milk Blueberries Orange Juice	Chickpea Chia Salad with Spring Greens Whole-grain Crackers Grapes Plant Milk	Chili de Verduras Tortilla Chips Spring Side Salad Mandarin Orange Plant Milk
Monday	Banana Muffin* 2-3 Prunes Orange Juice	Broccoli, Apple, Walnut Salad Quinoa Seasonal Fresh Fruit Medley Plant Milk	Artichokes with Hollandaise Sauce Whole-grain Roll Apple Chunks Plant Milk
Tuesday	Bagel with Seed Butter & Berries Orange Juice	Chickpea Chia Salad with Spring Greens* Whole-grain Crackers Grapes Plant Milk	Chili de Verduras* Tortilla Chips Spring Side Salad Mandarin Orange Plant Milk
Wednesday	Overnight Oats with Peaches Orange Juice	Broccoli, Apple, Walnut Salad* Quinoa Seasonal Fresh Fruit Medley Plant Milk	Vegetable Divan Whole-grain Bread Apple Chunks Plant Milk
Thursday	Bagel with Seed Butter & Berries Orange Juice	Butterbean & Corn Salad Whole-grain Chips or Crackers Grapes Plant Milk	Red & White Pizzas Garden Variety Salad Mandarin Orange Plant Milk
Friday	Overnight Oats with Peaches* Orange Juice	Crisp Vegetable & Hummus Sandwich Whole-grain Pita Wedges with extra Hummus Seasonal Fresh Fruit Medley Plant Milk	Vegetable Divan* Whole-grain Bread Apple Chunks Plant Milk
Saturday	Banana Muffin 2-3 Prunes Orange Juice	Butterbean & Corn Salad* Whole-grain Chips or Crackers Seasonal Fresh Fruit Medley Plant Milk	Red & White Pizzas* Garden Variety Salad Mandarin Orange Plant Milk

*Use leftovers to your advantage. Also, consider making double batches of items that freeze well to keep on hand.
To make planning easier, consider choosing just 2-3 breakfast or lunch items and rotate them for a week.
Include dry ready-to-eat whole-grain cereals that are good sources of iron and zinc in your breakfast rotation to help meet nutrient needs.
Use orange juice fortified with calcium and plant milk varieties that are fortified with protein (soymilk has equivalent levels of protein without requiring fortification) and calcium.
Veggie burgers or other ready-made plant-based foods may be added occasionally when preparation time is limited.

Weekly Menu Planner

	Breakfast	Lunch	Supper
Sunday			
Monday			
Tuesday			
Wednesday			
Thursday			
Friday			
Saturday			

Weekly Menu Planner

	Breakfast	Lunch	Supper
Sunday			
Monday			
Tuesday			
Wednesday			
Thursday			
Friday			
Saturday			

Weekly Menu Planner

	Breakfast	Lunch	Supper
Sunday			
Monday			
Tuesday			
Wednesday			
Thursday			
Friday			
Saturday			

	Breakfast	Lunch	Supper
Sunday			
Monday			
Tuesday			
Wednesday			
Thursday			
Friday			
Saturday			

Weekly Menu Planner

Appendix B
28 Days of Sample Meals and Nutrient Information

28 Days of Sample Meals

Tables 1 and 2 provide another resource to help you plan nutritionally sound meals. While each of the 28-days of meals in Table 1 are different, your personal menu may likely include the use of leftovers for convenience. Although, consuming the same food more than once in a given week is fine, it is important to recognize that foods vary in nutrient composition, so it is essential to eat a wide variety of foods in order to include all nutrients in your diet. Table 2 provides a general idea of the daily intake of nutrients that can be expected when following the sample meal plan in Table 1.

Table 1: 28 Days of Sample Meals

Day 1		Day 2	
Breakfast	Cal/Pro*	**Breakfast**	Cal/Pro*
1 Whole-grain Bagel with Seed Butter & Berries	513/17	1 large Banana Muffin	321/6
		3 Prunes	61/1
6 ounces Orange Juice	80/1	6 ounces Orange Juice	80/1
Lunch		**Lunch**	
1 cup Chickpea Chia Salad	318/10	1 cup Broccoli, Apple, Walnut Salad	217/4
1 cup Garden Salad Greens	12/1	½ cup Quinoa	111/4
8 Whole-grain Crackers	135/2	1 cup Blueberries	83/1
1 cup Grapes	62/1	½ cup Cooked Chickpeas	134/7
1 cup Unsweetened Soymilk	80/7	1 cup Unsweetened Soymilk	80/7
Supper		**Supper**	
1 Artichoke with Hollandaise Sauce	329/8	1 cup Down by the Bay Gumbo	171/6
1 Whole-grain Roll	75/2	1 Whole-grain French Roll	96/3
1 teaspoon Plant Butter	27/0	1 teaspoon Plant Butter	27/0
1 cup Seasonal Fresh Fruit Medley	65/1	1 medium Peach	59/1
1 cup Unsweetened Soymilk	80/7	1 cup Unsweetened Soymilk	80/7

*Cal/Pro = Calories and Protein (protein listed in grams)

(continues on next page)

Table 1: 28 Days of Sample Meals (continued)

Day 3		Day 4	
Breakfast	Cal/Pro*	**Breakfast**	Cal/Pro*
1 cup Dry Whole-grain Cereal such as Total®	140/3	1½ cups Overnight Oats with Peaches	309/8
1 cup Unsweetened Soymilk	80/7	6 ounces Orange Juice	80/1
1 small Banana	90/1		
Lunch		**Lunch**	
1 Crisp Vegetable & Hummus Sandwich	309/5	1 cup Lady Pea Salad	301/14
		1 cup Garden Salad Greens	12/1
1 Whole-grain Pita Bread (4" diameter)	75/3	1 Dill Pickle Spear	3/0
		8 Whole-grain Crackers	135/2
2½ tablespoons Classic Hummus	93/3	1 Orange (cut in slices)	62/1
1 cup Strawberry Halves	49/1	1 cup Unsweetened Soymilk	80/7
1 cup Unsweetened Soymilk	80/7		
Supper		**Supper**	
1 cup Chili de Verduras	245/12	1 cup Creamy Corn Chowder	188/8
8 Saltine Crackers	101/2	1 slice Whole-grain Bread	69/3
1 Spring Side Salad	153/2	1 teaspoon Plant Butter	27/0
1 small Apple	77/0	1 cup Grapes	62/1
1 cup Unsweetened Soymilk	80/7	1 cup Unsweetened Soymilk	80/7

*Cal/Pro = Calories and Protein (protein listed in grams)

(continues on next page)

Table 1: 28 Days of Sample Meals (continued)

Day 5		Day 6	
Breakfast	Cal/Pro*	**Breakfast**	Cal/Pro*
1 cup Good-Morning Grits ½ whole Tomato (cut in slices) ½ Grapefruit 6 ounces Orange Juice	201/3 11/1 51/1 80/1	1 cup Heavenly Hash Browns & ⅓ cup Black Beans 1 cup Mixed Salad Greens 1 tablespoon Poppy Seed Dressing 1 cup Chopped Cantaloupe 6 ounces Orange Juice	499/12 12/1 121/0 54/1 80/1
Lunch		**Lunch**	
1 cup Wild West Dip with Chips 1 cup Shredded Green Leaf Lettuce 1 cup Watermelon Chunks ¼ cup Pumpkin Seed Kernels 1 cup Unsweetened Soymilk	358/10 5/0 46/1 180/10 80/7	1 cup Quinoa Black Bean Bowl with Mango & Kale 1 cup Seasonal Fresh Fruit Medley 1 cup Unsweetened Soymilk	202/8 65/1 80/7
Supper		**Supper**	
1 Enchiladas Poblano ⅓ cup Black Beans ½ cup Pomegranate Arils 1 cup Unsweetened Soymilk	321/11 80/5 72/1 80/7	1 cup Broccoli & Potato Soup 1 slice 7-Grain Bread 1 teaspoon Plant Butter 1 cup Pineapple Chunks 1 cup Unsweetened Soymilk	149/7 84/4 27/0 82/1 80/7

*Cal/Pro = Calories and Protein (protein listed in grams)

(continues on next page)

Table 1: 28 Days of Sample Meals (continued)

Day 7	Cal/Pro*	Day 8	Cal/Pro*
Breakfast		**Breakfast**	
1⅓ cups Dry Cereal such as Multi-Grain Cheerios®	150/3	1 Whole-grain Bagel with Seed Butter & Berries	513/17
1 cup Unsweetened Soymilk	80/7	6 ounces Orange Juice	80/1
1 cup Strawberry Halves	49/1		
Lunch		**Lunch**	
1 cup Butter Bean & Corn Salad	289/10	1 cup Chickpea Chia Salad	318/10
8 Whole-grain Crackers	135/2	1 cup Garden Salad Greens	12/1
1 cup Sunshine Smoothie	100/3	8 Whole-grain Crackers	135/2
1 cup Unsweetened Soymilk	80/7	1 cup Grapes	62/1
		1 cup Unsweetened Soymilk	80/7
Supper		**Supper**	
2 Falafels with Tzatziki Sauce	332/7	1 cup French Market Soup	123/7
1 cup Cucumber Slices	16/1	1 slice Whole-grain Baguette	96/3
½ cup Quinoa	111/4	1 teaspoon Plant Butter	27/0
1 cup Pear Slices	94/1	1 cup Seasonal Fresh Fruit Medley	65/1
1 cup Unsweetened Soymilk	80/7	1 cup Unsweetened Soymilk	80/7

*Cal/Pro = Calories and Protein (protein listed in grams)

(continues on next page)

Table 1: 28 Days of Sample Meals (continued)

Day 9		Day 10	
Breakfast	Cal/Pro*	**Breakfast**	Cal/Pro*
1 cup Dry Whole-grain Cereal such as Total®	140/3	1 large Blueberry Muffin	305/5
		1 small Banana	90/1
1 cup Unsweetened Soymilk	80/7	6 ounces Orange Juice	80/1
3 Prunes	61/1		
Lunch		**Lunch**	
1 cup Broccoli, Apple, Walnut Salad	217/4	1 Crisp Vegetable & Hummus Sandwich	309/5
½ cup Quinoa	111/4		
1 cup Blueberries	83/1	1 Whole-grain Pita Bread (4"diameter)	75/3
1 cup Unsweetened Soymilk	80/7		
		2½ tablespoons Classic Hummus	93/3
		1 cup Strawberry Halves	49/1
		1 cup Unsweetened Soymilk	80/7
Supper		**Supper**	
1 Garden Wrap	438/14	¹⁄₁₂ Lasagna Vegetali	213/8
¼ Avocado	72/1	1 slice Whole-grain Ciabatta Bread	150/3
1 medium Peach	59/1	1 teaspoon Plant Butter	27/0
1 cup Unsweetened Soymilk	80/7	1 Spring Side Salad	153/2
		1 small Apple	77/0
		1 cup Unsweetened Soymilk	80/7

*Cal/Pro = Calories and Protein (protein listed in grams)

(continues on next page)

Table 1: 28 Days of Sample Meals (continued)

Day 11		Day 12	
Breakfast	Cal/Pro*	**Breakfast**	Cal/Pro*
1½ cups Overnight Oats with Peaches	309/8	1⅓ cups Dry Cereal such as Multi-Grain Cheerios®	150/3
6 ounces Orange Juice	80/1	1 cup Unsweetened Soymilk	80/7
		¼ cup Walnut Halves	164/4
		½ Grapefruit	51/1
Lunch		**Lunch**	
1 cup Lady Pea Salad	301/14	1 cup Wild West Dip with Chips	358/10
1 cup Garden Salad Greens	12/1	1 cup Shredded Green Leaf Lettuce	5/0
1 Dill Pickle Spear	3/0	1 cup Watermelon Chunks	46/1
8 Whole-grain Crackers	135/2	¼ cup Pumpkin Seed Kernels	180/10
1 Orange (cut in slices)	62/1	1 cup Unsweetened Soymilk	80/7
1 cup Unsweetened Soymilk	80/7		
Supper		**Supper**	
1 Lemongrass Ginger Vegetables & Tofu Noodle Bowl	366/20	1 Lentilly Sandwich	270/12
		½ cup Super Slaw	89/1
1 Spring Roll	156/4	½ cup Pomegranate Arils	72/1
1 cup Grapes	62/1	1 cup Unsweetened Soymilk	80/7
1 cup Unsweetened Soymilk	80/7		

*Cal/Pro = Calories and Protein (protein listed in grams)

(continues on next page)

Table 1: 28 Days of Sample Meals (continued)

Day 13		Day 14	
Breakfast	**Cal/Pro***	**Breakfast**	**Cal/Pro***
1 cup Heavenly Hash Browns & ⅓ cup Black Beans	499/12	3 Perfect Pancakes (includes fruit) 6 ounces Orange Juice	412/8 80/1
1 cup Mixed Salad Greens	12/1		
1 tablespoon Poppy Seed Dressing	121/0		
1 cup Chopped Cantaloupe	54/1		
6 ounces Orange Juice	80/1		
Lunch		**Lunch**	
1 cup Quinoa Black Bean Bowl with Mango & Kale	202/8	1 cup Butter Bean & Corn Salad 8 Whole-grain Crackers	289/10 135/2
1 cup Seasonal Fresh Fruit Medley	65/1	1 cup Strawberry Dream Smoothie	100/4
1 cup Unsweetened Soymilk	80/7	1 cup Unsweetened Soymilk	80/7
Supper		**Supper**	
1 cup Magnificent Macaroni Casserole	320/11	1 Night on the Mediterranean Gyro ½ cup Tabouli Salad	448/11 114/4
1 cup Garden Salad Greens	12/1	1 cup Pear Slices	94/1
2 tablespoons Italian Dressing	71/0	1 cup Unsweetened Soymilk	80/7
1 cup Pineapple Chunks	82/1		
1 cup Unsweetened Soymilk	80/7		

*Cal/Pro = Calories and Protein (protein listed in grams)

(continues on next page)

Table 1: 28 Days of Sample Meals (continued)

Day 15	Cal/Pro*	Day 16	Cal/Pro*
Breakfast		**Breakfast**	
1 Whole-grain Bagel with Seed Butter & Berries	513/17	1 large Banana Muffin	321/6
		3 Prunes	61/1
6 ounces Orange Juice	80/1	6 ounces Orange Juice	80/1
Lunch		**Lunch**	
1 cup Chickpea Chia Salad	318/10	1 cup Broccoli, Apple, Walnut Salad	217/4
1 cup Garden Salad Greens	12/1	½ cup Quinoa	111/4
8 Whole-grain Crackers	135/2	1 cup Blueberries	83/1
1 cup Grapes	62/1	1 cup Unsweetened Soymilk	80/7
1 cup Unsweetened Soymilk	80/7		
Supper		**Supper**	
1 cup Old Fashioned Squash Casserole	306/7	2 slices Red & White Pizzas	455/16
		1 Spring Side Salad	153/2
½ cup Fresh Field Peas	140/7	1 medium Peach	59/1
1 cup Seasonal Fresh Fruit Medley	65/1	1 cup Unsweetened Soymilk	80/7
1 cup Unsweetened Soymilk	80/7		

*Cal/Pro = Calories and Protein (protein listed in grams)

(continues on next page)

Table 1: 28 Days of Sample Meals (continued)

Day 17		Cal/Pro*	Day 18	Cal/Pro*
Breakfast			**Breakfast**	
1 cup Dry Whole-grain Cereal such as Total®		140/3	1½ cups Overnight Oats with Peaches	309/8
1 cup Unsweetened Soymilk		80/7	6 ounces Orange Juice	80/1
¼ cup Pumpkin Seed Kernels		180/10		
1 small Banana		90/1		
Lunch			**Lunch**	
1 Crisp Vegetable & Hummus Sandwich		309/5	1 cup Lady Pea Salad	301/14
			1 cup Garden Salad Greens	12/1
1 Whole-grain Pita Bread (4"diameter)		75/3	1 Dill Pickle Spear	3/0
			8 Whole-grain Crackers	135/2
2½ tablespoons Classic Hummus		93/3	1 Orange (cut in slices)	62/1
1 cup Strawberry Halves		49/1	1 cup Unsweetened Soymilk	80/7
1 cup Unsweetened Soymilk		80/7		
Supper			**Supper**	
1 cup Favorite Red Beans & Rice		234/9	1 serving Savory Spaghetti	408/17
1 Whole-grain French Roll		96/3	1 Spring Side Salad	153/2
1 teaspoon Plant Butter		27/0	1 slice Garlic Bread	150/4
1 small Apple		77/0	1 cup Grapes	62/1
1 cup Unsweetened Soymilk		80/7	1 cup Unsweetened Soymilk	80/7

*Cal/Pro = Calories and Protein (protein listed in grams)

(continues on next page)

Table 1: 28 Days of Sample Meals (continued)

Day 19		Day 20	
Breakfast	Cal/Pro*	**Breakfast**	Cal/Pro*
1 cup Good-Morning Grits	201/3	1⅓ cups Dry Cereal such as Multi-Grain Cheerios®	150/3
½ whole Tomato (cut in slices)	11/1		
½ Grapefruit	51/1	1 cup Unsweetened Soymilk	80/7
6 ounces Orange Juice	80/1	¼ cup Walnut Halves	164/4
		1 cup Chopped Cantaloupe	54/1
Lunch		**Lunch**	
1 cup Wild West Dip with Chips	358/10	1 cup Quinoa Black Bean Bowl with Mango & Kale	202/8
1 cup Shredded Green Leaf Lettuce	5/0		
1 cup Watermelon Chunks	46/1	1 cup Seasonal Fresh Fruit Medley	65/1
1 cup Unsweetened Soymilk	80/7	¼ cup Pumpkin Seed Kernels	180/10
		1 cup Unsweetened Soymilk	80/7
Supper		**Supper**	
1 serving Sesame Garlic Vegetables & Tofu with Rice	449/22	1 cup Simple Leek Soup	259/7
		1 slice Whole-grain Bread	69/3
1 Spring Roll	156/4	1 teaspoon Plant Butter	27/0
½ cup Pomegranate Arils	72/1	1 cup Pineapple Chunks	82/1
1 cup Unsweetened Soymilk	80/7	1 cup Unsweetened Soymilk	80/7

*Cal/Pro = Calories and Protein (protein listed in grams)

(continues on next page)

Table 1: 28 Days of Sample Meals (continued)

Day 21		Day 22	
Breakfast	**Cal/Pro***	**Breakfast**	**Cal/Pro***
3 Perfect Pancakes (includes fruit) 6 ounces Orange Juice	412/8 80/1	1 Whole-grain Bagel with Seed Butter & Berries 6 ounces Orange Juice	513/17 80/1
Lunch		**Lunch**	
1 cup Butter Bean & Corn Salad 8 Whole-grain Crackers 1 cup Sunshine Smoothie 1 cup Unsweetened Soymilk	289/10 135/2 100/3 80/7	1 cup Chickpea Chia Salad 1 cup Garden Salad Greens 8 Whole-grain Crackers 1 cup Grapes 1 cup Unsweetened Soymilk	318/10 12/1 135/2 62/1 80/7
Supper		**Supper**	
1 cup Southern Black-eyed Peas ½ whole Tomato (cut in slices) 1 Meltaway Cornbread Muffin 1 teaspoon Plant Butter 1 cup Pear Slices 1 cup Unsweetened Soymilk	150/9 11/1 188/2 27/0 94/1 80/7	$\frac{1}{12}$ slice Spiced Beanloaf 1 cup Parsley Mashed Potatoes ½ cup Buttered Sweet Peas 1 cup Seasonal Fresh Fruit Medley 1 cup Unsweetened Soymilk	171/8 195/4 76/4 65/1 80/7

*Cal/Pro = Calories and Protein (protein listed in grams)

(continues on next page)

Table 1: 28 Days of Sample Meals (continued)

Day 23		Day 24	
Breakfast	Cal/Pro*	**Breakfast**	Cal/Pro*
1 cup Dry Whole-grain Cereal such as Total®	140/3	1 large Blueberry Muffin	305/5
1 cup Unsweetened Soymilk	80/7	1 small Banana	90/1
¼ cup Walnut Halves	164/4	6 ounces Orange Juice	80/1
3 Prunes	61/1		
Lunch		**Lunch**	
1 cup Broccoli, Apple, Walnut Salad	217/4	1 Crisp Vegetable & Hummus Sandwich	309/5
½ cup Quinoa	111/4	1 Whole-grain Pita Bread (4" diameter)	75/3
1 cup Blueberries	83/1	2½ tablespoons Classic Hummus	93/3
1 cup Unsweetened Soymilk	80/7	1 cup Strawberry Halves	49/1
		1 cup Unsweetened Soymilk	80/7
Supper		**Supper**	
⅛ Spinach & Red Pepper Quiche	226/7	1 cup Split Pea & Carrot Soup	190/13
1 Spring Side Salad	153/2	1 Whole-grain Roll	75/2
1 medium Peach	59/1	1 teaspoon Plant Butter	27/0
1 cup Unsweetened Soymilk	80/7	1 small Apple	77/0
		1 cup Unsweetened Soymilk	80/7

*Cal/Pro = Calories and Protein (protein listed in grams)

(continues on next page)

Table 1: 28 Days of Sample Meals (continued)

Day 25		Day 26	
Breakfast	Cal/Pro*	**Breakfast**	Cal/Pro*
1½ cups Overnight Oats with Peaches	309/8	1⅓ cups Dry Cereal such as Multi-Grain Cheerios®	150/3
6 ounces Orange Juice	80/1	1 cup Unsweetened Soymilk	80/7
		½ Grapefruit	51/1
Lunch		**Lunch**	
1 cup Lady Pea Salad	301/14	1 cup Wild West Dip with Chips	358/10
1 cup Garden Salad Greens	12/1	1 cup Shredded Green Leaf Lettuce	5/0
1 Dill Pickle Spear	3/0	1 cup Watermelon Chunks	46/1
8 Whole-grain Crackers	135/2	¼ cup Pumpkin Seed Kernels	180/10
1 Orange (cut in slices)	62/1	1 cup Unsweetened Soymilk	80/7
1 cup Unsweetened Soymilk	80/7		
Supper		**Supper**	
2 Tasty Tacos	583/20	1 serving Topside Pot Pie	328/10
1 cup Grapes	62/1	1 cup Garden Salad Greens	12/1
1 cup Unsweetened Soymilk	80/7	2 tablespoons Italian Dressing	71/0
		½ cup Pomegranate Arils	72/1
		1 cup Unsweetened Soymilk	80/7

*Cal/Pro = Calories and Protein (protein listed in grams)

(continues on next page)

Table 1: 28 Days of Sample Meals (continued)

Day 27		Day 28	
Breakfast	Cal/Pro*	**Breakfast**	Cal/Pro*
1 cup Heavenly Hash Browns & ⅓ cup Black Beans	499/12	3 Perfect Pancakes (includes fruit)	412/8
1 cup Mixed Salad Greens	12/1	6 ounces Orange Juice	80/1
1 tablespoon Poppy Seed Dressing	121/0		
1 cup Chopped Cantaloupe	54/1		
6 ounces Orange Juice	80/1		
Lunch		**Lunch**	
1 cup Quinoa Black Bean Bowl with Mango & Kale	202/8	1 cup Butter Bean & Corn Salad	289/10
1 cup Seasonal Fresh Fruit Medley	65/1	8 Whole-grain Crackers	135/2
1 cup Unsweetened Soymilk	80/7	1 cup Strawberry Dream Smoothie	100/4
		1 cup Unsweetened Soymilk	80/7
Supper		**Supper**	
1 cup Turnip Greens & Dumplings	123/3	1 serving Vegetable Divan	312/9
½ cup Fresh Field Peas	140/7	½ cup Brown Rice	108/3
1 cup Pineapple Chunks	82/1	1 cup Pear Slices	94/1
1 cup Unsweetened Soymilk	80/7	1 cup Unsweetened Soymilk	80/7

*Cal/Pro = Calories and Protein (protein listed in grams)

Nutrient Information

Table 2 provides a general idea of the daily intake of nutrients that can be expected when following the suggested meal plan in Table 1. Table 2 lists the average, minimum, and maximum daily amounts of key nutrients that would be consumed over a set of 28 days of eating the meals which are specified in Table 1. The estimates are made assuming that only one serving of each item is consumed. Individual intake levels will vary with the number of servings, other foods consumed, as well as whether or not ingredients chosen contain fortification of certain nutrients. For more information about fortified nutrients, see **Chapters 6** and **8**. **Chapters 7** and **8** contain tips for obtaining additional protein or other nutrients of concern as needed.

Table 2 Mean (minimum, maximum) values of daily nutrient intake from the 28 days of sample meals detailed in Table 1

Calories	1,651 (1,427, 2,043)	Vitamin D micrograms*	10 (6, 17)
Protein grams	57 (47, 75)	Vitamin B12 micrograms*	7 (5, 11)
Carbohydrate grams	232 (168, 302)	Choline milligrams*	119 (70, 171)
Fiber grams	38 (29, 52)	Iodine micrograms*	46 (7, 97)
Fat grams	62 (45, 80)	Iron milligrams*	19 (12, 33)
Saturated Fat grams	10 (6, 13)	Zinc milligrams*	10 (4, 18)
Sodium milligrams	1,822 (1,092, 2,544)	Potassium milligrams*	3,365 (2,757, 4,235)
Calcium milligrams*	1,384 (1,162, 1,916)	Phosphorus milligrams*	1,138 (826, 1,555)

*Asterisks indicate nutrients for which the values were not available for all food items in the sample meals which may result in underreporting of the mean, (minimum, maximum) daily intake of those nutrients.

These estimates assume the use of iodized salt, orange juice fortified with calcium, as well as plant milk varieties that are fortified with calcium, vitamin B12, vitamin D, and protein (soymilk has equivalent levels of protein without requiring fortification).

Recipe and food calculations are approximations made by a registered dietitian nutritionist using NutriBase 19 Pro + Edition, v.19.1 (CyberSoft, Inc.), food manufacturers, or the USDA Agricultural Research Service Food Data Central.

Appendix C
Recipe Nutrient Estimations:
calcium, vitamin D, vitamin B12, iodine, iron,
zinc, choline, potassium, phosphorus

This section estimates the expected nutritional values for nine important nutrients from each recipe in this book. Because some data was missing, the nutrient values presented here for the nine nutrients are estimates representing the minimum amount of each nutrient that can be expected from consuming one serving of each recipe. Also, these estimates assume the use of iodized salt, as well as plant milk varieties that are fortified with calcium, vitamin B12, and vitamin D. Note that the nutrient values for the complete meals in which these recipes are used will be increased (variably) by the additional foods that are selected and included in each meal.

Supper

1. **Artichokes with Hollandaise Sauce—Nutrients Per Serving:** 89 milligrams calcium, 0 micrograms vitamin D, 0 micrograms vitamin B12, 0 micrograms iodine, 3 milligrams iron, 1 milligram zinc, 56 milligrams choline, 729 milligrams potassium, 192 milligrams phosphorus. Iodized salt and olive oil used in water for artichokes were not included in estimations.
2. **Broccoli and Potato Soup—Nutrients Per Serving:** 89 milligrams calcium, 1 microgram vitamin D, 1 microgram vitamin B12, 13 micrograms iodine, 2 milligrams iron, 1 milligram zinc, 30 milligrams choline, 503 milligrams potassium, 115 milligrams phosphorus
3. **Chili de Verduras—Nutrients Per Serving:** 130 milligrams calcium, 0 micrograms vitamin D, 0 micrograms vitamin B12, 20 micrograms iodine, 5 milligrams iron, 2 milligrams zinc, 36 milligrams choline, 996 milligrams potassium, 206 milligrams phosphorus

4. **Creamy Corn Chowder—Nutrients Per Serving:** 117 milligrams calcium, 4 micrograms vitamin D, 1 microgram vitamin B12, 8 micrograms iodine, 2 milligrams iron, 1 milligram zinc, 2 milligrams choline, 281 milligrams potassium, 102 milligrams phosphorus
5. **Down by the Bay Gumbo—Nutrients Per Serving:** 59 milligrams calcium, 0 micrograms vitamin D, 0 micrograms vitamin B12, 11 micrograms iodine, 2 milligrams iron, 1 milligram zinc, 28 milligrams choline, 402 milligrams potassium, 130 milligrams phosphorus
6. **Enchiladas Poblano—Nutrients Per Serving:** 151 milligrams calcium, 2 micrograms vitamin D, <1 microgram vitamin B12, 13 micrograms iodine, 3 milligrams iron, 1 milligram zinc, 36 milligrams choline, 652 milligrams potassium, 216 milligrams phosphorus
7. **Falafels with Tzatziki Sauce—Nutrients Per Serving:** 103 milligrams calcium, 2 micrograms vitamin D, <1 microgram vitamin B12, 37 micrograms iodine, 2 milligrams iron, 1 milligram zinc, 26 milligrams choline, 281 milligrams potassium, 118 milligrams phosphorus
8. **Favorite Red Beans and Rice—Nutrients Per Serving:** 59 milligrams calcium, 0 micrograms vitamin D, 0 micrograms vitamin B12, 3 micrograms iodine, 3 milligrams iron, 1 milligram zinc, 12 milligrams choline, 566 milligrams potassium, 215 milligrams phosphorus
9. **French Market Soup—Nutrients Per Serving:** 50 milligrams calcium, 0 micrograms vitamin D, 0 micrograms vitamin B12, 10 micrograms iodine, 2 milligrams iron, 1 milligram zinc, 27 milligrams choline, 546 milligrams potassium, 132 milligrams phosphorus
10. **Garden Wrap—Nutrients Per Serving:** 276 milligrams calcium, 0 micrograms vitamin D, 0 micrograms vitamin B12, 17 micrograms iodine, 4 milligrams iron, 1 milligram zinc, 8 milligrams choline, 467 milligrams potassium, 136 milligrams phosphorus
11. **Lasagna Vegetali—Nutrients Per Serving:** 87 milligrams calcium, <1 microgram vitamin D, <1 microgram vitamin B12, 17 micrograms iodine, 3 milligrams iron, 1 milligram zinc, 48 milligrams choline, 588 milligrams potassium, 109 milligrams phosphorus
12. **Lemongrass Ginger Vegetables and Tofu Noodle Bowl—Nutrients Per Serving:** 724 milligrams calcium, 0 micrograms vitamin D, 0 micrograms vitamin B12, 34 micrograms iodine, 4 milligrams iron, 2 milligrams zinc, 14 milligrams choline, 505 milligrams potassium, 230 milligrams phosphorus
13. **Lentillies—Nutrients Per Serving:** 102 milligrams calcium, <1 microgram vitamin D, <1 microgram vitamin B12, 0 micrograms iodine, 4 milligrams iron, 2 milligrams zinc, 20 milligrams choline, 537 milligrams potassium, 171 milligrams phosphorus
14. **Magnificent Macaroni Casserole—Nutrients Per Serving:** 196 milligrams calcium, 3 micrograms vitamin D, 1 microgram vitamin B12, 27 micrograms iodine, 3 milligrams iron, 2 milligrams zinc, 19 milligrams choline, 298 milligrams potassium, 159 milligrams phosphorus
15. **Night on the Mediterranean Gyro—Nutrients Per Serving:** 149 milligrams calcium, <1 microgram vitamin D, <1 microgram vitamin B12, 25 micrograms iodine, 2 milligrams iron, <1 milligram zinc, 16 milligrams choline, 357 milligrams potassium, 70 milligrams phosphorus
16. **Old Fashioned Squash Casserole—Nutrients Per Serving:** 120 milligrams calcium, 1 microgram vitamin D, <1 microgram vitamin B12, 8 micrograms iodine, 2 milligrams iron, 1 milligram zinc, 33 milligrams choline, 582 milligrams potassium, 123 milligrams phosphorus
17. **Red and White Pizzas—Nutrients Per Serving:** 158 milligrams calcium, 1 microgram vitamin D, <1 microgram vitamin B12, 59 micrograms iodine, 6 milligrams iron, 2 milligrams zinc, 3 milligrams choline, 374 milligrams potassium, 210 milligrams phosphorus

18. **Savory Spaghetti—Nutrients Per Serving:** 189 milligrams calcium, <1 microgram vitamin D, <1 microgram vitamin B12, 6 micrograms iodine, 5 milligrams iron, 3 milligrams zinc, 46 milligrams choline, 934 milligrams potassium, 318 milligrams phosphorus
19. **Sesame Garlic Vegetables and Tofu with Rice—Nutrients Per Serving:** 739 milligrams calcium, 0 micrograms vitamin D, 0 micrograms vitamin B12, 0 micrograms iodine, 5 milligrams iron, 3 milligrams zinc, 21 milligrams choline, 690 milligrams potassium, 392 milligrams phosphorus
20. **Simple Leek Soup—Nutrients Per Serving:** 241 milligrams calcium, 6 micrograms vitamin D, 1 microgram vitamin B12, 0 micrograms iodine, 3 milligrams iron, 1 milligram zinc, 39 milligrams choline, 541 milligrams potassium, 135 milligrams phosphorus
21. **Southern Black-eyed Peas—Nutrients Per Serving:** 13 milligrams calcium, 0 micrograms vitamin D, 0 micrograms vitamin B12, 0 milligrams iodine, 3 milligrams iron, <1 milligram zinc, 5 milligrams choline, 538 milligrams potassium, 21 milligrams phosphorus
22. **Spiced Beanloaf—Nutrients Per Serving:** 43 milligrams calcium, <1 microgram vitamin D, <1 microgram vitamin B12, 11 milligrams iodine, 2 milligrams iron, 1 milligram zinc, 12 milligrams choline, 290 milligrams potassium, 107 milligrams phosphorus
23. **Spinach and Sweet Pepper Quiche—Nutrients Per Serving:** 181 milligrams calcium, 2 micrograms vitamin D, <1 microgram vitamin B12, 17 micrograms iodine, 2 milligrams iron, 1 milligram zinc, 21 milligrams choline, 249 milligrams potassium, 101 milligrams phosphorus
24. **Split Pea and Carrot Soup—Nutrients Per Serving:** 37 milligrams calcium, 0 micrograms vitamin D, 0 micrograms vitamin B12, 4 micrograms iodine, 2 milligrams iron, 2 milligrams zinc, 50 milligrams choline, 566 milligrams potassium, 195 milligrams phosphorus
25. **Tasty Tacos—Nutrients Per Serving:** 138 milligrams calcium, 0 micrograms vitamin D, 0 micrograms vitamin B12, 17 micrograms iodine, 5 milligrams iron, 3 milligrams zinc, 68 milligrams choline, 1,329 milligrams potassium, 376 milligrams phosphorus
26. **Topside Pot Pie—Nutrients Per Serving:** 183 milligrams calcium, 5 micrograms vitamin D, 1 microgram vitamin B12, 25 micrograms iodine, 3 milligrams iron, 1 milligram zinc, 45 milligrams choline, 597 milligrams potassium, 168 milligrams phosphorus
27. **Turnip Greens and Dumplings—Nutrients Per Serving:** 151 milligrams calcium, 1 microgram vitamin D, 0 micrograms vitamin B12, 13 micrograms iodine, 2 milligrams iron, <1 milligram zinc, 2 milligrams choline, 199 milligrams potassium, 103 milligrams phosphorus
28. **Vegetable Divan—Nutrients Per Serving:** 245 milligrams calcium, 2 micrograms vitamin D, <1 microgram vitamin B12, 4 micrograms iodine, 2 milligrams iron, 1 milligram zinc, 21 milligrams choline, 657 milligrams potassium, 191 milligrams phosphorus

Sides

1. **Buttered Sweet Peas—Nutrients Per Serving:** 16 milligrams calcium, 0 micrograms vitamin D, 0 micrograms vitamin B12, 8 milligrams iodine, 1 milligram iron, 1 milligram zinc, 19 milligrams choline, 111 milligrams potassium, 59 milligrams phosphorus
2. **Classic Hummus—Nutrients Per Serving:** 49 milligrams calcium, 0 micrograms vitamin D, 0 micrograms vitamin B12, 34 micrograms iodine, 2 milligrams iron, 1 milligram zinc, 28 milligrams choline, 206 milligrams potassium, 133 milligrams phosphorus

3. **Meltaway Cornbread—Nutrients Per Serving:** 125 milligrams calcium, 1 microgram vitamin D, <1 microgram vitamin B12, 6 milligrams iodine, 1 milligram iron, <1 milligram zinc, 2 milligrams choline, 51 milligrams potassium, 140 milligrams phosphorus
4. **Parsley Mashed Potatoes—Nutrients Per Serving:** 91 milligrams calcium, 2 micrograms vitamin D, <1 microgram vitamin B12, 39 milligrams iodine, 2 milligrams iron, 1 milligram zinc, 24 milligrams choline, 842 milligrams potassium, 112 milligrams phosphorus
5. **Sauteed Asparagus—Nutrients Per Serving:** 6 milligrams calcium, 0 micrograms vitamin D, 0 micrograms vitamin B12, 4 micrograms iodine, 1 milligram iron, <1 milligram zinc, 4 milligrams choline, 48 milligrams potassium, 12 milligrams phosphorus
6. **Seasonal Fresh Fruit Medley—Nutrients Per Serving:** 15 milligrams calcium, 0 micrograms vitamin D, 0 micrograms vitamin B12, 0 milligrams iodine, <1 milligram iron, <1 milligram zinc, 10 milligrams choline, 313 milligrams potassium, 22 milligrams phosphorus
7. **Spring Side Salad—Nutrients Per Serving:** 31 milligrams calcium, 0 micrograms vitamin D, 0 micrograms vitamin B12, 0 micrograms iodine, 1 milligram iron, <1 milligram zinc, 8 milligrams choline, 342 milligrams potassium, 45 milligrams phosphorus
8. **Super Slaw—Nutrients Per Serving:** 23 milligrams calcium, 0 micrograms vitamin D, 0 micrograms vitamin B12, 4 micrograms iodine, <1 milligram iron, <1 milligram zinc, 6 milligrams choline, 100 milligrams potassium, 15 milligrams phosphorus
9. **Tabouli Salad—Nutrients Per Serving:** 35 milligrams calcium, 0 micrograms vitamin D, 0 micrograms vitamin B12, 4 micrograms iodine, 2 milligrams iron, 1 milligram zinc, 21 milligrams choline, 235 milligrams potassium, 96 milligrams phosphorus

Lunch

1. **Broccoli, Apple, Walnut Salad—Nutrients Per Serving:** 46 milligrams calcium, 0 micrograms vitamin D, 0 micrograms vitamin B12, 14 micrograms iodine, 1 milligram iron, 1 milligram zinc, 24 milligrams choline, 315 milligrams potassium, 103 milligrams phosphorus
2. **Butter Bean and Corn Salad—Nutrients Per Serving:** 56 milligrams calcium, 0 micrograms vitamin D, 0 micrograms vitamin B12, 34 micrograms iodine, 3 milligrams iron, 1 milligram zinc, 5 milligrams choline, 798 milligrams potassium, 168 milligrams phosphorus
3. **Chickpea Chia Salad—Nutrients Per Serving:** 88 milligrams calcium, 0 micrograms vitamin D, 0 micrograms vitamin B12, 7 micrograms iodine, 3 milligrams iron, 2 milligrams zinc, 50 milligrams choline, 469 milligrams potassium, 214 milligrams phosphorus
4. **Crisp Vegetables and Hummus Sandwich—Nutrients Per Serving:** 192 milligrams calcium, 0 micrograms vitamin D, 0 micrograms vitamin B12, 8 micrograms iodine, 2 milligrams iron, 1 milligram zinc, 15 milligrams choline, 245 milligrams potassium, 56 milligrams phosphorus
5. **Lady Pea Salad—Nutrients Per Serving:** 48 milligrams calcium, 0 micrograms vitamin D, <1 microgram vitamin B12, 34 micrograms iodine, 5 milligrams iron, 2 milligrams zinc, 57 milligrams choline, 515 milligrams potassium, 273 milligrams phosphorus
6. **Quinoa Black Bean Bowl with Mango and Kale—Nutrients Per Serving:** 49 milligrams calcium, 0 micrograms vitamin D, 0 micrograms vitamin B12, 13 micrograms iodine, 2 milligrams iron, 1 milligram zinc, 16 milligrams choline, 420 milligrams potassium, 169 milligrams phosphorus

7. **Wild West Dip with Chips—Nutrients Per Serving:** 74 milligrams calcium, 0 micrograms vitamin D, <1 microgram vitamin B12, 18 micrograms iodine, 3 milligrams iron, 2 milligrams zinc, 30 milligrams choline, 538 milligrams potassium, 204 milligrams phosphorus

Breakfast

1. **Bagels with Seed Butter and Berries—Nutrients Per Serving:** 70 milligrams calcium, 0 micrograms vitamin D, 0 micrograms vitamin B12, 0 micrograms iodine, 5 milligrams iron, 3 milligrams zinc, 18 milligrams choline, 488 milligrams potassium, 396 milligrams phosphorus
2. **Banana Muffins—Nutrients Per Serving:** 100 milligrams calcium, 0 micrograms vitamin D, 0 micrograms vitamin B12, 11 micrograms iodine, 1 milligram iron, 1 milligram zinc, 7 milligrams choline, 229 milligrams potassium, 224 milligrams phosphorus
3. **Blueberry Muffins—Nutrients Per Serving:** 141 milligrams calcium, 1 microgram vitamin D, <1 microgram vitamin B12, 11 micrograms iodine, 1 milligram iron, 1 milligram zinc, 5 milligrams choline, 122 milligrams potassium, 220 milligrams phosphorus
4. **Good-Morning Grits—Nutrients Per Serving:** 86 milligrams calcium, 2 micrograms vitamin D, 0 micrograms vitamin B12, 14 micrograms iodine, 1 milligram iron, <1 milligram zinc, 14 milligrams choline, 184 milligrams potassium, 60 milligrams phosphorus
5. **Heavenly Hash Browns and Black Beans—Nutrients Per Serving:** 136 milligrams calcium, 0 micrograms vitamin D, 0 micrograms vitamin B12, 0 micrograms iodine, 3 milligrams iron, 1 milligram zinc, 11 milligrams choline, 959 milligrams potassium, 204 milligrams phosphorus
6. **Overnight Oats with Peaches—Nutrients Per Serving:** 406 milligrams calcium, 1 microgram vitamin D, 0 micrograms vitamin B12, 17 micrograms iodine, 10 milligrams iron, 1 milligram zinc, 15 milligrams choline, 571 milligrams potassium, 370 milligrams phosphorus
7. **Perfect Pancakes or Waffles—Nutrients Per Serving:** 329 milligrams calcium, 1 microgram vitamin D, 0 micrograms vitamin B12, 34 micrograms iodine, 2 milligrams iron, 1 milligram zinc, 16 milligrams choline, 282 milligrams potassium, 403 milligrams phosphorus

Beverages

1. **Strawberry Dream Smoothie—Nutrients Per Serving:** 143 milligrams calcium, 1 microgram vitamin D, 1 microgram vitamin B12, 0 micrograms iodine, 1 milligram iron, <1 milligram zinc, 10 milligrams choline, 395 milligrams potassium, 62 milligrams phosphorus
2. **Sunshine Smoothie—Nutrients Per Serving:** 146 milligrams calcium, 1 microgram vitamin D, 1 microgram vitamin B12, 0 micrograms iodine, 1 milligram iron, <1 milligram zinc, 12 milligrams choline, 380 milligrams potassium, 58 milligrams phosphorus

Desserts

1. **Apple Crisp—Nutrients Per Serving:** 112 milligrams calcium, 2 micrograms vitamin D, 0 micrograms vitamin B12, 0 micrograms iodine, 2 milligrams iron, <1 milligram zinc, 9 milligrams choline, 200 milligrams potassium, 131 milligrams phosphorus
2. **Chocolate Chip Oatmeal Cookies—Nutrients Per Serving:** 22 milligrams calcium, 1 microgram vitamin D, 0 micrograms vitamin B12, 8 micrograms iodine, 1 milligram iron, <1 milligram zinc, 1 milligram choline, 51 milligrams potassium, 51 milligrams phosphorus

Notes

Chapter 1: Introduction

1. Le LT, Sabaté J. Beyond meatless, the health effects of vegan diets: findings from the Adventist cohorts. *Nutrients*. 2014;6(6):2131-2147.
2. Melina V, Craig W, Levin S. Position of the Academy of Nutrition and Dietetics: vegetarian diets. *J Acad Nutr Diet*. 2016;116(12):1970-1980.
3. Qian F, Liu G, Hu FB, Bhupathiraju SN, Sun Q. Association between plant-based dietary patterns and risk of type 2 diabetes: a systematic review and meta-analysis. *JAMA Intern Med*. 2019;179(10):1335-1344.
4. Kahleova H, Petersen KF, Shulman GI, et al. Effect of a low-fat vegan diet on body weight, insulin sensitivity, postprandial metabolism, and intramyocellular and hepatocellular lipid levels in overweight adults: a randomized clinical trial. *JAMA Netw Open*. 2020;3(11):e2025454.
5. Barnard ND, Cohen J, Jenkins DJ, et al. A low-fat vegan diet improves glycemic control and cardiovascular risk factors in a randomized clinical trial in individuals with type 2 diabetes. *Diabetes Care*. 2006;29(8):1777-1783.
6. Huang J, Liao LM, Weinstein SJ, Sinha R, Graubard BI, Albanes D. Association between plant and animal protein intake and overall and cause-specific mortality. *JAMA Intern Med*. 2020;180(9):1173-1184.
7. Kim H, Caulfield LE, Garcia-Larsen V, Steffen LM, Coresh J, Rebholz CM. Plant-based diets are associated with a lower risk of incident cardiovascular disease, cardiovascular disease mortality, and all-cause mortality in a general population of middle-aged adults. *J Am Heart Assoc*. 2019;8(16):e012865.

8. Papier K, Fensom GK, Knuppel A, et al. Meat consumption and risk of 25 common conditions: outcome-wide analyses in 475,000 men and women in the UK Biobank study. *BMC Medicine*. 2021;19(1):53.
9. National Cancer Institute. Chemicals in Meat Cooked at High Temperatures and Cancer Risk. National Cancer Institute at the National Institutes of Health website. Reviewed July 11, 2017. Last accessed June 17, 2022. https://www.cancer.gov/about-cancer/causes-prevention/risk/diet/cooked-meats-fact-sheet.
10. World Cancer Research Fund International/American Institute for Cancer Research. Diet, nutrition, physical activity and colorectal cancer. Continuous Update Project Report: Colorectal Cancer 2018. Last accessed June 17, 2022. https://www.wcrf.org/dietandcancer/colorectal-cancer/.
11. Barnard ND, Alwarith J, Rembert E, et al. A Mediterranean diet and low-fat vegan diet to improve body weight and cardiometabolic risk factors: a randomized, cross-over trial. *J Am Coll Nutr*. 2021;1-13.
12. Kim SJ, de Souza RJ, Choo VL, et al. Effects of dietary pulse consumption on body weight: a systematic review and meta-analysis of randomized controlled trials. *Am J Clin Nutr*. 2016;103(5):1213-1223.
13. Ikizler TA, Burrowes JD, Byham-Gray LD, et al. KDOQI clinical practice guideline for nutrition in CKD: 2020 update. *Am J Kidney Dis*. 2020, 76(3)(suppl 1):S1-S107.
14. Rodriguiz A. RDN Resources for Professionals: Plant-based Diets in Chronic Kidney Disease. Vegetarian Nutrition a dietetic practice group of the Academy of Nutrition and Dietetics website. Reviewed by Melissa Prest. Last accessed June 17, 2022. https://www.vndpg.org.
15. Reynolds AN, Akerman AP, Mann J. Dietary fibre and whole-grains in diabetes management: Systematic review and meta-analyses. *PLoS Medicine*. 2020;17(3): e1003053.
16. Tomova A, Bukovsky I, Rembert E, et al. The effects of vegetarian and vegan diets on gut microbiota. *Front Nutr*. 2019;6:47.
17. Rooks MG, Garrett WS. Gut microbiota, metabolites and host immunity. *Nat Rev Immunol*. 2016;16(6):341-352.
18. Lazar V, Ditu LM, Pircalabioru GG, et al. Aspects of gut microbiota and immune system interactions in infectious diseases, immunopathology, and cancer. *Front Immunol*. 2018;9:1830.
19. David LA, Maurice CF, Carmody RN, et al. Diet rapidly and reproducibly alters the human gut microbiome. *Nature*. 2014;505(7484):559-563.
20. Glick-Bauer M, Yeh M. The health advantage of a vegan diet: exploring the gut microbiota connection. *Nutrients*. 2014;6(11):4822-4838.

21. Dahl WJ, Stewart ML. Position of the Academy of Nutrition and Dietetics: health implications of dietary fiber. *J Acad Nutr Diet*. 2015;115(11):1861-1870.
22. Lattimer JM, Haub MD. Effects of dietary fiber and its components on metabolic health. *Nutrients*. 2010;2(12):1266-1289.

Chapter 2: Nutrition Basics

1. Institute of Medicine. *Dietary Reference Intakes for Energy, Carbohydrate, Fiber, Fat, Fatty Acids, Cholesterol, Protein, and Amino Acids (Macronutrients)*. The National Academies Press; 2005. https://www.nap.edu.
2. Melina V, Craig W, Levin S. Position of the Academy of Nutrition and Dietetics: vegetarian diets. *J Acad Nutr Diet*. 2016;116(12):1970-1980.
3. Office of Dietary Supplements. Calcium: Fact Sheet for Health Professionals. Office of Dietary Supplements at the National Institutes of Health website. Updated June 2, 2022. Last accessed June 17, 2022. https://ods.od.nih.gov/factsheets/Calcium-HealthProfessional/.
4. Office of Dietary Supplements. Vitamin D: Fact Sheet for Health Professionals. Office of Dietary Supplements at the National Institutes of Health website. Updated June 2, 2022. Last accessed June 17, 2022. https://ods.od.nih.gov/factsheets/VitaminD-HealthProfessional/.
5. Office of Dietary Supplements. Vitamin B12: Fact Sheet for Health Professionals. Office of Dietary Supplements at the National Institutes of Health website. Updated March 9, 2022. Last accessed June 17, 2022. https://ods.od.nih.gov/factsheets/VitaminB12-HealthProfessional/.
6. Pawlak R. RDN Resources for Professionals: Vitamin B12 in Vegetarian Diets. Vegetarian Nutrition a dietetic practice group of the Academy of Nutrition and Dietetics website. Updated by Chris Vogliano. Last accessed June 17, 2022. https://www.vndpg.org.
7. Office of Dietary Supplements. Iodine: Fact Sheet for Health Professionals. Office of Dietary Supplements at the National Institutes of Health website. Updated April 28, 2021. Last accessed June 17, 2022. https://ods.od.nih.gov/factsheets/Iodine-HealthProfessional/.
8. Office of Dietary Supplements. Iron: Fact Sheet for Health Professionals. Office of Dietary Supplements at the National Institutes of Health website. Updated April 5, 2022. Last accessed June 17, 2022. https://ods.od.nih.gov/factsheets/Iron-HealthProfessional/.
9. Office of Dietary Supplements. Zinc: Fact Sheet for Health Professionals. Office of Dietary Supplements at the National Institutes of Health website. Updated December 7, 2021. Last accessed June 17, 2022. https://ods.od.nih.gov/factsheets/Zinc-HealthProfessional/.

10. Norris J. RDN Resources for Professionals: Zinc in Vegetarian Diets. Vegetarian Nutrition a dietetic practice group of the Academy of Nutrition and Dietetics website. Updated by Lauren Panoff. Last accessed June 17, 2022. https://www.vndpg.org.
11. Office of Dietary Supplements. Choline: Fact Sheet for Health Professionals. Office of Dietary Supplements at the National Institutes of Health website. Updated June 2, 2022. Last accessed June 17, 2022. https://ods.od.nih.gov/factsheets/Choline-HealthProfessional/.
12. Norris, J. RDN Resources for Professionals: Choline in Vegetarian Diets. Vegetarian Nutrition a dietetic practice group of the Academy of Nutrition and Dietetics website. Updated by Chris Vogliano. Last accessed June 17, 2022. https://www.vndpg.org.
13. Office of Dietary Supplements. Omega-3 Fatty Acids: Fact Sheet for Health Professionals. Office of Dietary Supplements at the National Institutes of Health website. Updated June 2, 2022. Last accessed June 17, 2022. https://ods.od.nih.gov/factsheets/Omega3FattyAcids-HealthProfessional/.
14. Davis B, Melina V. *Becoming Vegan: Comprehensive Edition*. Book Publishing Co; 2014.
15. Mangels R, Messina V, Messina M. *The Dietitian's Guide to Vegetarian Diets.* 3rd ed. Jones & Bartlett Learning; 2011.

Chapter 3: Meal Planning for a Plant-Based Diet

1. Larson, E. RD Resources for Professionals: Sports Nutrition for Vegetarians. Vegetarian Nutrition a dietetic practice group of the Academy of Nutrition and Dietetics website. Last accessed June 17, 2022. https://www.vndpg.org.
2. Mangels, R. RDN Resources for Professionals: Vegetarian Nutrition for School-Aged Children. The Academy of Nutrition and Dietetics Vegetarian Nutrition Dietetic Practice Group website. Updated by Karla Moreno-Bryce. Last accessed June 17, 2022. https://www.vndpg.org.
3. Kharod, P. RD Resources for Consumers: Vegetarian/Vegan Teens. Vegetarian Nutrition a dietetic practice group of the Academy of Nutrition and Dietetics website. Last accessed June 17, 2022. https://www.vndpg.org.

Chapter 4: Tips for Success

1. Carruth BR, Ziegler PJ, Gordon A, Barr SI. Prevalence of picky eaters among infants and toddlers and their caregivers' decisions about offering a new food. *J Am Diet Assoc.* 2004;104(1 Suppl 1):s57-s64.
2. Satter E. *Child of Mine Feeding with Love and Good Sense*. Bull Publishing Company. 2000.

3. Mangels, R. RDN Resources for Professionals: Vegetarian Nutrition for Toddlers and Preschoolers. Vegetarian Nutrition a dietetic practice group of the Academy of Nutrition and Dietetics website. Updated by Lauren Panoff. Last accessed June 17, 2022. https://www.vndpg.org.
4. Mangels, R. RDN Resources for Professionals: Vegetarian Nutrition for School-Aged Children. Vegetarian Nutrition a dietetic practice group of the Academy of Nutrition and Dietetics website. Updated by Karla Moreno-Bryce. Last accessed June 17, 2022. https://www.vndpg.org.

Chapter 5: Planning for Snacks and Desserts

1. Centers for Disease Control and Prevention. Choking Hazards. Centers for Disease Control and Prevention website. Page last reviewed February 25, 2022. Last accessed June 17, 2022. https://www.cdc.gov/nutrition/InfantandToddlerNutrition/foods-and-drinks/choking-hazards.html.

Chapter 6: Beverages

1. Stipanuk MH, Caudill MA. *Biochemical, Physiological, and Molecular Aspects of Human Nutrition*. 3rd ed. Saunders Elsevier; 2013.
2. National Institute of Diabetes and Digestive and Kidney Diseases. Bladder Infection (Urinary Tract Infection) in Adults. National Institute of Diabetes and Digestive and Kidney Diseases at the National Institutes of Health website. Reviewed March 2017. Last accessed June 17, 2022. https://www.niddk.nih.gov/health-information/urologic-diseases/bladder-infection-uti-in-adults/all-content.
3. Mayo Clinic Staff. Urinary Tract Infection (UTI). Mayo Clinic website. Last accessed June 17, 2022.
http://www.mayoclinic.org/diseases-conditions/urinary-tract-infection/basics/lifestyle-home-remedies/con-20037892.
4. Mahan LK, Raymond JL. *Krause's Food and the Nutrition Care Process*. 14th ed. Elsevier; 2017.
5. Institute of Medicine. *Dietary Reference Intakes for Water, Potassium, Sodium, Chloride, and Sulfate*. The National Academies Press; 2005. https://www.nap.edu/.
6. Nutritional values were obtained from the U.S. Department of Agriculture, Agricultural Research Service. FoodData Central, 2019. Last accessed June 17, 2022. https://fdc.nal.usda.gov/, or from food manufacturers.
7. American Academy of Pediatrics. Fruit Juice and Your Child's Diet. The AAP Parenting website – HealthyChildren.org. Updated May 22, 2017. Last accessed June 17, 2022.

https://www.healthychildren.org/English/healthy-living/nutrition/Pages/Fruit-Juice-and-Your-Childs-Diet.aspx.
8. Institute of Medicine. *Dietary Reference Intakes: The Essential Guide to Nutrient Requirements*. The National Academies Press; 2006. https://www.nap.edu/.

Chapter 7: Protein Matters

1. Institute of Medicine. *Dietary Reference Intakes for Energy, Carbohydrate, Fiber, Fat, Fatty Acids, Cholesterol, Protein, and Amino Acids (Macronutrients)*. The National Academies Press; 2005. https://www.nap.edu/.
2. Melina V, Craig W, Levin S. Position of the Academy of Nutrition and Dietetics: vegetarian diets. *J Acad Nutr Diet*. 2016;116(12):1970-1980.
3. U.S. Department of Agriculture and U.S. Health and Human Services. *Dietary Guidelines for Americans, 2020-2025*. 9th Edition. U.S. Department of Agriculture and U.S. Health and Human Services; 2020. https://www.dietaryguidelines.gov/.
4. Yanez E, Uauy R, Zacarias I, Barrera G. Long-term validation of 1 g of protein per kilogram body weight from a predominantly vegetable mixed diet to meet the requirements of young adult males. *J Nutr*. 1986; 116(5):865-872.
5. Davis B, Melina V. *Becoming Vegan: Comprehensive Edition*. Book Publishing Co; 2014.
6. Mangels R, Messina V, Messina M. *The Dietitian's Guide to Vegetarian Diets*. 3rd ed. Jones & Bartlett Learning; 2011.
7. Palmer, S. RDN Resources for Professionals: Protein in Vegetarian and Vegan Diets. Vegetarian Nutrition a dietetic practice group of the Academy of Nutrition and Dietetics website. Last accessed June 17, 2022. https://www.vndpg.org.
8. Norris J. Protein and Amino Acids. Vegan Health website. Updated February 2020. Last accessed June 17, 2022. https://veganhealth.org/.
9. Bhasin S, Apovian CM, Travison TG, et al. Effect of protein intake on lean body mass in functionally limited older men: a randomized clinical trial. *JAMA Intern Med*. 2018;178(4):530-541.
10. Bauer J, Biolo G, Cederholm T, et al. Evidence-based recommendations for optimal dietary protein intake in older people: a position paper from the PROT-AGE Study Group. *J Am Med Dir Assoc*. 2013;14(8):542-559.
11. Deutz NE, Bauer JM, Barazzoni R, et al. Protein intake and exercise for optimal muscle function with aging: recommendations from the ESPEN Expert Group. *Clin Nutr*. 2014;33(6):929-936.
12. Thomas DT, Erdman KA, Burke LM. Position of the Academy of Nutrition and Dietetics, Dietitians of Canada, and the American College of Sports Medicine: nutrition and athletic performance. *J Acad Nutr Diet*. 2016;116(3):501-528.

13. Nutritional values were obtained from the U.S. Department of Agriculture, Agricultural Research Service. FoodData Central, 2019. Last accessed June 17, 2022. https://fdc.nal.usda.gov/, or from food manufacturers.

Chapter 8: Nutrients of Concern and Summary Chart

Calcium

1. Office of Dietary Supplements. Calcium: Fact Sheet for Health Professionals. Office of Dietary Supplements at the National Institutes of Health website. Updated June 2, 2022. Last accessed June 17, 2022. https://ods.od.nih.gov/factsheets/Calcium-HealthProfessional/.
2. Messina, Virginia. RD Resources for Professionals: Meeting Calcium Recommendations on a Vegan Diet. Vegetarian Nutrition a dietetic practice group of the Academy of Nutrition and Dietetics website. Updated by Lauren Panoff. Last accessed June 17, 2022. https://www.vndpg.org.
3. U.S. Department of Agriculture, Agricultural Research Service. FoodData Central, 2019. Last accessed June 17, 2022. https://fdc.nal.usda.gov/.

Vitamin D

1. Office of Dietary Supplements. Vitamin D: Fact Sheet for Health Professionals. Office of Dietary Supplements at the National Institutes of Health website. Updated June 2, 2022. Last accessed June 17, 2022. https://ods.od.nih.gov/factsheets/VitaminD-HealthProfessional/.
2. Nutritional values were obtained from the U.S. Department of Agriculture, Agricultural Research Service. FoodData Central, 2019. Last accessed June 17, 2022. https://fdc.nal.usda.gov/, or from food manufacturers.

Vitamin B12

1. Office of Dietary Supplements. Vitamin B12: Fact Sheet for Health Professionals. Office of Dietary Supplements at the National Institutes of Health website. Updated March 9, 2022. Last accessed June 17, 2022. https://ods.od.nih.gov/factsheets/VitaminB12-HealthProfessional/.
2. Melina V, Craig W, Levin S. Position of the Academy of Nutrition and Dietetics: Vegetarian Diets. *J Acad Nutr Diet*. 2016;116(12):1970-1980.

3. Pawlak R. RDN Resources for Professionals: Vitamin B12 in Vegetarian Diets. Vegetarian Nutrition a dietetic practice group of the Academy of Nutrition and Dietetics website. Updated by Chris Vogliano. Last accessed June 17, 2022. https://www.vndpg.org.
4. Institute of Medicine. *Dietary Reference Intakes: The Essential Guide to Nutrient Requirements.* The National Academies Press; 2006. https://www.nap.edu/.
5. Stipanuk MH, Caudill MA. *Biochemical, Physiological, and Molecular Aspects of Human Nutrition.* 3rd ed. Saunders Elsevier; 2013.
6. Bor MV, von Castel-Roberts KM, Kauwell GP, et al. Daily intake of 4 to 7 micrograms dietary vitamin B-12 is associated with steady concentrations of vitamin B-12-related biomarkers in a healthy young population. *Am J Clin Nutr.* 2010; 91(3):571-577.
7. EFSA NDA Panel (EFSA Panel on Dietetic Products, Nutrition and Allergies), 2015. Scientific Opinion on Dietary Reference Values for cobalamin (vitamin B12). EFSA Journal 2015;13(7):4150, 64pp.
8. Carmel R. How I treat cobalamin (vitamin B12) deficiency. *Blood.* 2008; 112(6):2214-2221.
9. Nutritional values were obtained from the U.S. Department of Agriculture, Agricultural Research Service. FoodData Central, 2019. Last accessed June 17, 2022. https://fdc.nal.usda.gov/, or from food manufacturers.

Iodine

1. Office of Dietary Supplements. Iodine: Fact Sheet for Health Professionals. Office of Dietary Supplements at the National Institutes of Health website. Updated April 28, 2021. Last accessed June 17, 2022. https://ods.od.nih.gov/factsheets/Iodine-HealthProfessional/.
2. U.S. Department of Agriculture, Agricultural Research Service. FoodData Central, 2019. Last accessed June 17, 2022. https://fdc.nal.usda.gov/.

Iron

1. Office of Dietary Supplements. Iron: Fact Sheet for Health Professionals. Office of Dietary Supplements at the National Institutes of Health website. Updated April 5, 2022. Last accessed June 17, 2022. https://ods.od.nih.gov/factsheets/Iron-HealthProfessional/.
2. Melina V, Craig W, Levin S. Position of the Academy of Nutrition and Dietetics: vegetarian diets. *J Acad Nutr Diet.* 2016;116(12):1970-1980.
3. Messina, V. Nutritional and health benefits of dried beans. *Am J Clin Nutr.* 2014; 100 Suppl 1:437S-42S.
4. Centers for Disease Control and Prevention. Recommendations to prevent and control iron deficiency in the United States . *MMWR Recomm Rep.* 1998;47(RR-3):1-29.

5. Norris, J. RDN Resources for Consumers: Iron in Vegetarian Diets. Vegetarian Nutrition a dietetic practice group of the Academy of Nutrition and Dietetics website. Updated by Chris Vogliano. Last accessed June 17, 2022. https://www.vndpg.org.
6. Thomas DT, Erdman KA, Burke LM. American College of Sports Medicine Joint Position Statement. nutrition and athletic performance. *Med Sci Sports Exerc*. 2016;48(3):543-568.
7. Davis B, Melina V. *Becoming Vegan: Comprehensive Edition*. Book Publishing Co; 2014.
8. Mahan LK, Raymond JL. *Krause's Food and the Nutrition Care Process*. 14th ed. Elsevier; 2017.
9. Stipanuk MH, Caudill MA. *Biochemical, Physiological, and Molecular Aspects of Human Nutrition*. 3rd ed. Saunders Elsevier; 2013.
10. Institute of Medicine *Dietary Reference Intakes for Vitamin A, Vitamin K, Arsenic, Boron, Chromium, Copper, Iodine, Iron, Manganese, Molybdenum, Nickel, Silicon, Vanadium, and Zinc*. The National Academies Press. 2001. https://www.nap.edu.
11. Norris, J. RDN Resources for Professionals: Iron in Vegetarian Diets. Vegetarian Nutrition a dietetic practice group of the Academy of Nutrition and Dietetics website. Updated by Chris Vogliano. Last accessed June 17, 2022. https://www.vndpg.org.
12. Nutritional values were obtained from the U.S. Department of Agriculture, Agricultural Research Service. FoodData Central, 2019. Last accessed June 17, 2022. https://fdc.nal.usda.gov/, or from food manufacturers.

Zinc

1. Office of Dietary Supplements. Zinc: Fact Sheet for Health Professionals. Office of Dietary Supplements at the National Institutes of Health website. Updated December 7, 2021. Last accessed June 17, 2022. https://ods.od.nih.gov/factsheets/Zinc-HealthProfessional/.
2. Mangels R, Messina V, Messina M. *The Dietitian's Guide to Vegetarian Diets*. 3rd ed. Jones & Bartlett Learning; 2011.
3. Melina V, Craig W, Levin S. Position of the Academy of Nutrition and Dietetics: vegetarian diets. *J Acad Nutr Diet*. 2016;116(12):1970-1980.
4. Davis B, Melina V. *Becoming Vegan: Comprehensive Edition*. Book Publishing Co; 2014.
5. Mangels R. *The Everything Vegan Pregnancy Book*. Adams Media; 2011.
6. Messina, V. Nutritional and health benefits of dried beans. *Am J Clin Nutr*. 2014; 100 Suppl 1:437S-42S.
7. Norris J. RDN Resources for Consumers: Zinc in Vegetarian Diets. Vegetarian Nutrition a dietetic practice group of the Academy of Nutrition and Dietetics website. Updated by Lauren Panoff. Last accessed June 17, 2022. https://www.vndpg.org.
8. Institute of Medicine. *Dietary Reference Intakes: The Essential Guide to Nutrient Requirements.* The National Academies Press; 2006. https://www.nap.edu/.

9. Nutritional values were obtained from the U.S. Department of Agriculture, Agricultural Research Service. FoodData Central, 2019. Last accessed June 17, 2022. https://fdc.nal.usda.gov/, or from food manufacturers.

Choline

1. Office of Dietary Supplements. Choline: Fact Sheet for Health Professionals. Office of Dietary Supplements at the National Institutes of Health website. Updated June 2, 2022. Last accessed June 17, 2022.
https://ods.od.nih.gov/factsheets/Choline-HealthProfessional/.
2. Norris, J. RDN Resources for Professionals: Choline in Vegetarian Diets. Vegetarian Nutrition a dietetic practice group of the Academy of Nutrition and Dietetics website. Updated by Chris Vogliano. Last accessed June 17, 2022. https://www.vndpg.org.
3. U.S. Department of Agriculture, Agricultural Research Service. FoodData Central, 2019. Last accessed June 17, 2022. https://fdc.nal.usda.gov/.

Omega 3 Fatty Acids

1. Office of Dietary Supplements. Omega-3 Fatty Acids: Fact Sheet for Health Professionals. Office of Dietary Supplements at the National Institutes of Health website. Updated June 2, 2022. Last accessed June 17, 2022.
https://ods.od.nih.gov/factsheets/Omega3FattyAcids-HealthProfessional/.
2. Vogliano, C. RDN Resources for Professionals: Omega-3 Fatty Acids and Vegetarian Diets. Vegetarian Nutrition a dietetic practice group of the Academy of Nutrition and Dietetics website. Reviewed by Jack Norris. Last accessed June 17, 2022. https://www.vndpg.org.
3. Mozaffarian D, Appel LJ, Van Horn L. Components of a cardioprotective diet: new insights. *Circulation.* 2011;123(24):2870-2891.
4. Ratnayake WM, Galli C. Fat and fatty acid terminology, methods of analysis and fat digestion and metabolism: a background review paper. *Ann Nutr Metab*. 2009;55(1-3):8-43.
5. Weiser MJ, Butt CM, Mohajeri MH. Docosahexaenoic acid and cognition throughout the lifespan. *Nutrients*. 2016;8(2):99.
6. Melina V, Craig W, Levin S. Position of the Academy of Nutrition and Dietetics: vegetarian diets. *J Acad Nutr Diet*. 2016;116(12):1970-1980.
7. Burns-Whitmore B, Froyen E, Heskey C, et. al. Alpha-linolenic and linoleic fatty acids in the vegan diet: do they require Dietary Reference Intake/Adequate Intake special consideration? *Nutrients*. 2019;11(10):2365.

8. Lane KE, Wilson M, Hellon TG, Davies IG. Bioavailability and conversion of plant-based sources of omega-3 fatty acids - a scoping review to update supplementation options for vegetarians and vegans. *Crit Rev Food Sci Nutr*. 2021;1-16.
9. U.S. Food and Drug Administration and U.S. Environmental Protection Agency. Eating Fish: Advice about Eating Fish: For Women Who Are or Might Become Pregnant, Breastfeeding Mothers, and Young Children. U.S. Food & Drug Administration website. Revised October, 2021. Last accessed June 17, 2022. https://www.fda.gov/food/consumers/advice-about-eating-fish.
10. Nutritional values were obtained from the U.S. Department of Agriculture, Agricultural Research Service. FoodData Central, 2019. Last accessed June 17, 2022. https://fdc.nal.usda.gov/, or from food manufacturers.

Index

Amino acids, 6–7
Athletes
    iron, 45
    protein suggestions, 26
    snacks, 10–11, 17–18

Beans
    soaking methods, 68–69
Beverages, 177
    juice, 22
    Strawberry Dream Smoothie, 178
    Sunshine Smoothie, 179
    water, 21–24
Breakfast, 164
    Bagels with Seed Butter and Berries, 165
    Banana Muffins, 166–67
    Blueberry Muffins, 168–69
    Good-Morning Grits, 170–71
    Heavenly Hash Browns and Black Beans, 172–73
    Overnight Oats with Peaches, 174
    Perfect Pancakes or Waffles, 175–76

Calcium, 6–7, 9–10, 21–24, 62, 206–12
    oxalates, 35
    vitamin D, 36–38

Cancer, 3
Children
    serving sizes, 15
    snacks, 10–11, 17–18
    zinc, 50
Choline, 6–7, 55–58, 62, 206–12
Chop, 69
Chronic kidney disease, 4
Constipation, 4
Cooking terms
    chop, 69
    dice, 69
    julienne, 69
    mince, 69

Desserts, 17–19, 180
    Apple Crisp, 181–82
    Chocolate Chip Oatmeal Cookies, 183–84
Diabetes, type 2, 3
Dice, 69

Fiber, 4

Heart disease, 3

Immune system, 4

Inflammation, 4
Iodine, 6–7, 42–44, 62, 206–12
Iron, 6–7, 45–49, 62, 68, 206–12

Julienne, 69

Kidney disease, 4

Lectin, 68
Lunch, 152
    Broccoli, Apple, Walnut Salad, 153
    Butter Bean and Corn Salad, 154
    Chickpea Chia Salad, 155–56
    Crisp Vegetables and Hummus Sandwich, 157–58
    Lady Pea Salad, 159
    Quinoa Black Bean Bowl with Mango and Kale, 160–61
    Wild West Dip with Chips, 162–63

Main Meals. *See* Supper
Microbiome, 4
Mince, 69
Multivitamin, 63

Obesity, 4
Oligosaccharides, 68
Omega-3 fatty acids, 6–7, 59–62
    alpha-linolenic acid (ALA), 59–62
    docosahexaenoic acid (DHA), 59–62
    eicosapentaenoic acid (EPA), 59–62

Phosphorus, 206–12
Phytates, 45, 50, 68
Phytonutrients, 4
Plant-based
    definition, 5
Potassium, 206–12
Protein
    amino acids, 6–7
    athletes, 26
    older adults, 26

    pregancy, 26
Salads
    Broccoli, Apple, Walnut Salad, 153
    Butter Bean and Corn Salad, 154
    Chickpea Chia Salad, 155–56
    Lady Pea Salad, 159
    Spring Side Salad, 148–49
    Tabouli Salad, 151
Sides, 139
    Buttered Sweet Peas, 140
    Classic Hummus, 141–42
    Meltaway Cornbread, 143
    Parsley Mashed Potatoes, 144–45
    Sauteed Asparagus Spears, 146
    Seasonal Fresh Fruit Medley, 147
    Spring Side Salad, 148–49
    Super Slaw, 150
    Tabouli Salad, 151
Smoothies, 177
    Strawberry Dream Smoothie, 178
    Sunshine Smoothie, 179
Snacks, 17–19
Sodium, 206
Supper, 76
    Artichoke with Hollandaise Sauce, 77–78
    Broccoli and Potato Soup, 79–80
    Chili de Verduras, 81–82
    Creamy Corn Chowder, 83–84
    Down by the Bay Gumbo, 85–86
    Enchiladas Poblano, 87–89
    Falafels with Tzatziki Sauce, 90–92
    Favorite Red Beans and Rice, 93–94
    French Market Soup, 95–96
    Garden Wrap, 97–98
    Lasagna Vegetali, 99–101
    Lemongrass Ginger Vegetables and Tofu Noodle Bowl, 102–4
    Lentillies, 105–6
    Magnificent Macaroni Casserole, 107–8
    Night on the Mediterranean Gyro, 109–10
    Old Fashioned Squash Casserole, 111–12

Red and White Pizzas, 113–15
Savory Spaghetti, 116–17
Sesame Garlic Vegetables and Tofu with Rice, 118–20
Simple Leek Soup, 121–22
Southern Black-eyed Peas, 123
Spiced Beanloaf, 124–25
Spinach and Sweet Pepper Quiche, 126–28
Split Pea and Carrot Soup, 129
Tasty Tacos, 130–31
Topside Pot Pie, 132–34
Turnip Greens and Dumplings, 135–36
Vegetable Divan, 137–38

Teenagers
    snacks, 10–11, 17–18
Toxins, 4

Vegetarian
    lacto-ovo, 11
    pesco, 11
Vitamin B12, 6–7, 10, 39–41, 62, 206–12
Vitamin D, 6–7, 10, 36–38, 62, 206–12

Water, 21–24

Zinc, 6–7, 50–54, 62, 68, 206–12

www.ingramcontent.com/pod-product-compliance
Lightning Source LLC
Chambersburg PA
CBHW080411170426
43194CB00015B/2781